Hearing Care for the Older Adult

D1711090

Butterworth-Heinemann Series in Communications Disorders

Charlena M. Seymour, Ph.D., Series Editor

Battle, D.E. *Communication Disorders in Multicultural Populations* (1993)

Billeaud, F.P. *Communication Disorders in Infants and Toddlers: Assessment and Intervention* (1993)

Huntley, R.A., & Helfer, K.S. *Communication in Later Life* (1995)

Kricos, P.B., & Lesner, S.A. *Hearing Care for Older Adults: Audiologic Rehabilitation* (1995)

Maxon, A.B., & Brackett, D. *The Hearing-Impaired Child: Infancy Through High School Years* (1992)

Wall, L.G. *Hearing for the Speech-Language Pathologist and Health Care Professional* (1995)

Hearing Care for the Older Adult:

Audiologic Rehabilitation

Edited by

Patricia B. Kricos, Ph.D.
Professor of Communication Processes and Disorders
University of Florida
Gainesville

Sharon A. Lesner, Ph.D.
Professor of Audiology
School of Communicative Disorders
The University of Akron, Ohio

ELMHURST COLLEGE LIBRARY

JUN

2003

Butterworth–Heinemann
Boston Oxford Melbourne Singapore Toronto Munich New Delhi Tokyo

Copyright ©1995 by Butterworth-Heinemann

℞ A member of the Reed Elsevier group

All rights reserved.

No part of this publication may be reproduced, stored in a retrieval system, or transmitted in any form or by any means, electronic, mechanical, photocopying, recording, or otherwise, without the prior written permission of the publisher.

Every effort has been made to ensure that the drug dosage schedules within this text are accurate and conform to standards accepted at time of publication. However, as treatment recommendations vary in the light of continuing research and clinical experience, the reader is advised to verify drug dosage schedules herein with information found on product information sheets. This is especially true in cases of new or infrequently used drugs.

∞ Recognizing the importance of preserving what has been written, Butterworth-Heinemann prints its books on acid-free paper whenever possible.

Library of Congress Cataloging-in-Publication Data
Hearing Care for the older adult: audiologic rehabilitation / edited
    by Patricia B. Kricos, Sharon A. Lesner.
        p.   cm.   — (Butterworth–Heinemann series in communications
    disorders)
    Includes bilbiographical references and index.
    ISBN 0-7506-9531-5 (alk. paper)
    1. Aged, Deaf—Rehabilitation. I.Kricos, Patricia B. (Patricia
Bender), 1948- . II. Lesner, Sharon A., 1951- . III Series.
    [DNLM: 1. Hearing Disorders—in old age. 2. Hearing Disorders
—rehabilitation. 3. Rehabilitation—methods. 4. Rehabilitation—in
old age. WV 270 H433 1995]
RF291.5.A35H425   1995
618.97'789—dc20
DNLM/DLC
for Library of Congress   95-1130
                                                                    CIP

British Library Cataloguing-in-Publication Data
A catalogue record for this book is available from the British Library.

The publisher offers discounts on bulk orders of this book.
For information, please write:
Manager of Special Sales
Butterworth-Heinemann
313 Washington Street
Newton, MA 02158-1626

10 9 8 7 6 5 4 3 2

Printed in the United States of America

We dedicate this book to our grandmothers, Winifred Bender and Mary Andorka, whose unconditional love and support have always been there for us.

Contents

Contributing Authors

Judy Abrahamson, M.A.
Olin Teague Veterans Administration Medical Center, Temple, Texas
4. Effective and Relevant Programming

Alice E. Holmes, Ph.D.
Associate Professor of Audiology, Department of Communicative Disorders,
University of Florida
3. Hearing Aids and Older Adults

Mary Beth Jennings, M.C.I.Sc.
Aural Rehabilitation Audiologist, Department of Audiology and Speech
Pathology, The Canadian Hearing Society, Toronto, Ontario
*10. Service Delivery Models for Older Adults with Hearing Impairments:
Individual Sessions*

Patricia B. Kricos, Ph.D.
Professor of Communication Processes and Disorders, University of
Florida, Gainesville
*1. Characteristics of the Aged Population; 2. Audiologic Rehabilitation
Assessment: A Holistic Approach*

Sharon A. Lesner, Ph.D.
Professor of Audiology, School of Communicative Disorders
The University of Akron, Ohio
*2. Audiologic Rehabilitation Assessment: A Holistic Approach; 9. Group
Hearing Care for Older Adults*

Richmond B. Mowry, M.S., M.P.H.
Co-Owner, Professional Hearing Services—Littleton, Colorado
7. Older Adults in Long-Term Care Facilities

Sharon A. Sandridge, Ph.D.
Department of Otolaryngology and Communicative Disorders,
The Cleveland Clinic Foundation, Cleveland, Ohio
6. Beyond Hearing Aids: Use of Auxiliary Aids

Diane Shultz, M.A.
Practicing Audiologist, Sun City, Arizona
7. Older Adults in Long-Term Care Facilities

Robert M. Traynor, Ed.D.
Adjunct Professor of Audiology, Department of Communication Disorders,
University of Northern Colorado, Greeley; Clinical Professor of Audiology,
Department of Audiology, University of Colorado Health Sciences Center,
Denver
*8. Financial and Marketing Considerations in the Rehabilitation of Older
Adults*

Samuel Trychin, Ph.D.
Professor of Psychology, Gallaudet University, Washington, D.C.
5. Counseling Older Adults with Hearing Impairments

Preface

This book is dedicated to the fastest growing segment of the United States population, the elderly. The United States Bureau of the Census, in its projections of the United States population from 1982 until 2050, predicted a dramatic increase in the number of older adults in this country, and estimated that by the year 2025 approximately 58.6 million Americans will be 65 years of age or older; 19 percent of the population will be elderly. Although there is some conflict among studies of the prevalence of hearing loss among the elderly, it is generally accepted that close to half of all people 65 years of age and older have some degree of hearing loss.

The predicted increase in the next few decades in the number of elderly people in the United States, many of whom will have hearing impairments, has tremendous ramifications for the marketing of hearing care services for the elderly population. The purpose of this book is to present a practical, comprehensive, and viable model of service delivery to meet the needs of the elderly. The focus of the book is on audiologic rehabilitation of older adults with hearing impairments.

Because hearing loss has its most profound impact on communication, ultimately the primary goal of audiologic rehabilitation is to enable adults with hearing impairments to experience the least stressful communication possible, given constraints imposed by the hearing problem. The presence of hearing loss may have an impact on virtually all aspects of a person's lifestyle. The scope of audiologic rehabilitation must, therefore, extend beyond the enhancement of communication status. It is critical to determine how a hearing impairment may affect a person with a hearing impairment socially, emotionally, and, for some elderly adults, vocationally to provide effective and relevant services to reduce the handicap that may result from a hearing impairment.

Historically, audiologic rehabilitation (until recently more commonly referred to as aural rehabilitation) has been a vague and ill-defined entity, connoting images of lipreading and auditory training in some minds, hearing-aid fitting in others, and a required course or two taken by audiology students in still others. The demise of this concept of audiologic rehabilitation is ironic given that it was the rehabilitation component that, after World War II, gave rise to the field of audiology. At the cusp of a new century, it is encouraging to see a re-definition of audiologic rehabilitation, one that goes beyond lipreading and auditory training to include components such as psychosocial aspects of hearing impairment, hearing-aid orientation, assistive devices, programming for significant others, and emphasis on improving conversational and interactive skills.

Before 1974, audiologists made the strong argument to what was then their professional organization, the American Speech-Language-Hearing Association, that they needed to be able to dispense hearing aids in such a way that a comprehensive program, including the fitting of hearing aids and other audiologic rehabilitation services, could be provided to a client with a hearing impairment. It was a common notion at that time that an audiologist was a superior choice over a hearing-aid dealer to dispense hearing aids by virtue of the audiologist's ability to provide comprehensive services to the public, rather than just to dispense a hearing aid. Unfortunately, the focus in the private practice of audiology has been on dispensing hearing aids, rather than on organized, comprehensive programming for rehabilitation. The results of research for a master's thesis written by Linda Logan in 1990 at the University of Florida suggest that the differences between hearing-aid dealers and audiologists are not striking in the provision of rehabilitation programming. The audiologic rehabilitation of elderly people is a concept that has yet to be embraced in clinical practice despite the enthusiasm of a relatively small number of researchers and practitioners who have seen the benefits that can be reaped for both the elderly adult and the practitioner as a result of an organized, comprehensive approach to audiologic rehabilitation.

One of the problems frequently cited by audiologists in private practice is that providing comprehensive rehabilitation to elderly adults is not cost effective. A number of models of audiologic rehabilitation have been proposed, most of which have emanated from university training programs in which the bills are paid by the Board of Regents. One of the aims of this book is to provide realistic service-delivery models that can easily be implemented by private practitioners and that are economically feasible. Thus, we have assembled a group of chapter authors who represent a variety of practice settings, including Veterans Administration Medical Centers, private practices, hospitals, retirement homes, and corporate rehabilitation agencies. The service delivery models described in this book are based on two tenets: (1) every new user of a hearing aid needs and benefits from an organized program of audiologic rehabilitation that goes beyond a cursory explanation of how to use the hearing aid; and (2) the provision of comprehensive audiologic rehabilitation to older adults can be cost effective.

The latter tenet is something of which the authors are ever mindful as they present their philosophy throughout this book: audiologic rehabilitation is an indispensable part of the total treatment program of a person with a hearing impairment. The reader can be assured that the models presented in this book are not based on the availability of two graduate students for each elderly client, as might be the situation in a university clinic. A cost-benefit analysis of audiologic rehabilitation of elderly adults may yield a number of benefits beyond actual dollar profitability of service delivery. A practitioner who incorporates systematic, comprehensive audiologic rehabilitation into his or her practice may find a host of other benefits: satisfied customers, competent hearing aid users, good community relations, and, in our experience, the personal satisfaction of delivering the best possible services to the consumer. Audiologic rehabilitation of the elderly is challenging, yet it offers great professional rewards.

The first chapter of the book defines the characteristics of the older adult population, including general and audiologic characteristics. Subsequent chapters deal with identification of, evaluation of, and programming for the aged population. Extremely important are the final two chapters, which outline service delivery models for older adults with hearing impairments, including both group and individual programming suggestions. These final two chapters provide outlines of sessions that the practitioner can use as a reference and model. This book is addressed primarily to practicing audiologists, who may work in a variety of settings: private dispensing practice, medical center, or community speech and hearing center, to name a few. The book was written because of our perception of a void in the literature that deals with elderly people with hearing impairments. Above all, we have written this book because of our own optimism and confidence in the ability of the elderly to participate in and benefit from audiologic rehabilitation that is specifically designed to meet their needs.

P.B.K.
S.A.L.

Chapter 1

Characteristics of the Aged Population

Patricia B. Kricos

DEFINITIONS OF OLD AGE

Who are the elderly? This seemingly straightforward question is actually quite difficult to answer, because of the heterogeneity of the population. Conventional wisdom, based primarily on usual age of retirement, suggests that the elderly are people 65 years of age and older. Because this population is so varied, however, the 65-year-and-older convention is not an adequate benchmark for old age. As with the younger population, we can expect to see large individual differences among the elderly in a variety of attributes, and thus there is a danger of overgeneralizing their characteristics. Older people vary considerably in their health status, social and work activities, family situation, hearing abilities, and other important areas. Some elderly are still employed full-time; many are retired. Many are healthy; some are frail and confused and depend on the care of others. Most still live in a house or an apartment; only a small percentage live in a long-term care facility. Some have large incomes from savings, pensions, and investments; many depend primarily on Social Security benefits and have tight living budgets. Some have normal, in some cases near perfect, hearing, whereas many suffer from hearing handicaps that have a negative impact on their quality of life.

Is 55 years of age old? Is 75 years? Gerontology researchers have found it useful to consider older adults in subgroups. Neugarten (1975), for example, suggested that we conceptualize two groupings of elderly people: the young–old, ages 55 to 75 years, and the old–old, ages 75 years and older. Other researchers have provided even finer categorizations into smaller groupings such as the young–old (55 to 64 years), middle–old (65 to 74 years), and the old–old (75 years and older) (Botwinick, 1984; Silverman, 1987). The rationale for subdivision by specific age groups is that members of a particular age subgroup share more characteristics than would be the case if the more general 65 year-and-older convention were used. Piscopo (1985) categorized the older population not as much on the basis of age as on mental, emotional, and physical performance. His super–old group consisted of people who engage in a variety of physical and social activities, including master's competitions and marathons, and who bicycle, jog, play tennis and racquetball, and swim, among other activities. At the other end of Piscopo's age-wellness spectrum is the old–old, who are frail elders who are limited functionally in their mental, physical, emotional, and social capabilities. Using both age and wellness, Hooyman and Kiyak (1988) describe the *frisky* (ages 65 to 74 years), the *frail* (ages 75 to 85 years), and the *fragile* (older than 85 years). These authors acknowledge that there is still considerable diversity within these divisions.

In this book, the term *elderly* is used in general to refer to people who have reached their 65th birthday. Even with their great individual differences, older adults do have a great deal in common with each other. They possess some unique characteristics that separate them from the younger population. This chapter is devoted to delineation of some of these characteristics. An appreciation of both the physical (internal) changes and the social (external) changes experienced by older adults will increase the audiologist's likelihood of providing relevant services to this population.

DEMOGRAPHICS OF THE ELDERLY POPULATION

According to projections of population changes made by the United States Bureau of the Census in its 1988 report, at present, adults older than 65 years number approximately 31,559,000, more than 12 percent of the population. A huge increase is projected for the future—the Census Bureau predicts that there will be 39,362,000 older adults by the year 2010. Cunningham and Brookbank (1988) predict that the percentage of elderly is projected to be between 13 and 18 percent by the year 2020.

Korper (1989) noted that the rate of growth of the elderly population is projected to be somewhat greater after the year 2000 than during the 1990s. Between 1985 and 2000 the group 85 years and older will increase the most rapidly. Between the years 2000 and 2020, however, the 65- to 74-year group will increase the most rapidly, because the post–World War II baby boom generation will enter the elderly category. The proportion of elderly 85 years and older is projected to double, from 1.2 percent in 1985 to 2.4 percent in 2020. Not only will the absolute numbers of older adults increase, but also will the proportion of elderly that composes the general population.

Such dramatic changes in demographics will have considerable impact on the field of audiology. As will become even clearer from reading the section entitled "Prevalence of Hearing Loss in the Elderly" later in this chapter, the field of audiology has a challenge ahead in meeting the hearing health care needs of the elderly. The information in this book should provide a blueprint for designing effective and relevant audiologic rehabilitation services for the elderly population.

MYTHS ABOUT AGING

Stereotypes and misconceptions connected with aging abound. The elderly are frequently portrayed as frail, whiny, confused, depressed, troublesome, and senile. Even though the realities of aging do not fit the stereotypes, certain myths continue to be prevalent. A discussion of a few of these myths follows.

Myth: The elderly have trouble walking. Cox (1988) reported that 20 percent of people 65 years and older have trouble walking. Subscribers to this myth therefore fail to acknowledge the 80 percent of older people who have no trouble getting around.

Myth: The elderly experience difficulties in thinking clearly. True, Cox (1988) says, for 5 to 15 percent of aged people, but 85 to 95 percent of the elderly think clearly.

Myth: The elderly experience limitations in daily activities. According to research reported by Cox (1988), 60 to 90 percent of older people sampled had no limitation at all.

Myth: Old people are alienated from their families, especially from their children. Shanas (1980) reviewed a number of research studies that showed this myth is not true. In her own research, for example, Shanas found that three of four older adults who live alone had seen at least one of their children during the week before they were interviewed for the study.

Myth: The elderly typically have at least one disabling chronic condition. According to Atchley (1993), at least 60 percent of the elderly have no disabling condition.

Myth: Most of the elderly are institutionalized. According to Nussbaum et al (1989), only about 5 percent of the elderly are in nursing homes at any given time.

Myth: The elderly are senile. Approximately 4 percent of the elderly suffer from severe senility. No more than 15 percent suffer from senility of any degree, including mild mental disorders (Nussbaum et al, 1989).

This review of some of the more common myths associated with aging is not intended to deny the real problems that may accompany aging. Comparison of the myths with the realities, however, seems to indicate that the myths, rather than being based on complete falsehoods, for the main part are exaggerations of the problems experienced by the elderly. Cunningham and Brookbank (1988) reported that despite the prevalence of myths and misconceptions surrounding the elderly, most people, young and old alike, do not view the aged in a strongly negative way.

CHANGES THAT ACCOMPANY AGING

Atchley (1993) pointed out that aging is not one single process but many and that it has many possible outcomes, some positive and some negative. The previous section delineated some of the common misconceptions concerning aging and the older adult population. The purpose of this section is to outline some of the many changes that may accompany aging. These include physical, sensory, and, in the broad sense, psychologic changes such as changes in personality and lifestyle.

Physical Changes

Cox (1988) pointed out that for most people, aging carries some connotation of deterioration of health and vitality. Through numerous studies conducted by biologists it has been determined that physical aging can influence the functioning of the body in a number of ways. Hooyman and Kiyak (1988) pointed out that almost every organ system shows some decline with age in functional or reserve capacity. At 80 years of age, for example, the volume of oxygen that can be absorbed into the blood is only about half as much as at 40 years. In turn, this reduction in oxygen volume decreases the physical energy available to the body. Atchley (1993) suggested, however, that this decline in physical energy is not likely to interfere with typical social functioning.

Certain structural changes in the body may also take place as a result of aging. As they age, adults may become shorter, and the ability to move with ease may be affected. The latter may be due to joint stiffening, arthritis, or loss of muscle strength.

Physical appearance changes. Wrinkled skin, gray hair, age spots, baldness, and midriff bulge are common examples of the effects aging may have on appearance. Changes in the appearance and texture of skin and hair are often the most visible signs of aging.

Health may decline. The number of chronic conditions increases with age. The most frequently occurring chronic conditions that afflict older people include various forms of heart disease, hypertension, and different forms of arthritis (Hendricks & Hendricks, 1986). Many of these physical conditions, such as loss of teeth, are not necessarily disabling. Others, such as heart conditions and arthritis, may result in serious disability. Atchley (1993) noted that many health care professionals assume that a certain amount of disabling illness is normal for an aging person, and he strongly disagreed with this assumption. Although limiting chronic conditions are common among older people, many of these conditions are preventable and treatable, and all can be compensated for to some extent. Atchley (1993) therefore stated that limiting physical illness should be considered *atypical* of the older adult population. The wide variations in the degree of health experienced by the elderly can be accounted for by differences in diet, lifestyle, and, in large part, heredity.

The effects of aging on the central nervous system have been studied extensively. A decrease in brain weight, reduction in cerebral blood circulation, and atrophy and shrinkage of neurons have been well documented (Gioiella & Bevil, 1985). Age-related slowing of motor neuron conduction has been demonstrated with electromyography. The effects of age-related chemical and structural changes in the brain on human behavior are only beginning to be understood. Although there has been extensive documentation of the aging of the brain, there has been less focus on how age changes in the brain affect its capacity to react to its complex internal and external environments.

Many experiments have been conducted to investigate the speed with which people of varying ages can perform certain tasks. These studies almost always have found that older people, on the average, are slower to respond than younger people. Cunningham and Brookbank (1988), however, point out that conclusions based on group averages may be misleading because they do not account for the large individual differences among both the young and the old. Examination of data from individual people reveals that some young people are slow and some old people are fast, and there is a danger in overgeneralizing.

Other forms of biologic aging have been noted for the urinary system, the gastrointestinal system, and sexuality. Extensive coverage of age changes in human organ systems is provided in a number of gerontology texts—Cox (1988); Cunningham and Brookbank (1988); Hendricks and Hendricks (1986); Kart (1994); Schaie and Geiwitz (1982).

The undeniable physiologic changes and chronic conditions that may accompany aging need to be recognized and taken into consideration by audiologists who provide services to older adults. Equally important to keep in mind, however, is that despite having one or more chronic conditions, approximately 80 percent of older Americans lead full lives and pursue daily activities. Even in the presence of a limiting condition, most older adults, when asked to compare their health with that of others their age, report they are in as good or better health than most of their friends and are not prevented from doing most of the things they want to do (Cox, 1988). Acknowledging the prevalent chronic conditions that may accompany aging, then, does not mean expecting an older person to assume the role of a sick, frail, and feeble person.

Sensory Changes

The importance of the sensory processes for maintaining contact and interacting with the world cannot be overestimated. The literature on the effects of aging on sensory and perceptual abilities is extensive. Because this book deals specifically with older people with hearing impairments, an entire section is devoted later in this chapter to describing their hearing difficulties. This section on sensory changes that accompany aging briefly delineates changes that may accompany sensory mechanisms other than the auditory channel.

Vision

An important sensory ability to consider in the context of hearing impairment is vision, which may be affected through senescence in a number of ways. Visual acuity, as measured by devices such as Snellen charts and Titmus vision screeners, is the first characteristic of vision that comes to mind when most people consider the visual problems of the elderly. Up to the age of 40 to 50 years, little change in acuity is noted, but after that time there may be a marked decline. By the age of 70 years, without correction, poor vision is the rule rather than the exception (Botwinick, 1984). Atchley (1993), however, pointed out that even though decreases in visual acuity may be the norm, what should be of most interest to professionals who work with the elderly is actual functional vision. From data he collected on Ohio drivers, Atchley concluded that if one looks at *corrected* vision, by age of 60 years, more than 90 percent of older adults are still visually qualified for unrestricted driving; at the age of 80 years, 70 percent are still qualified. Atchley also observed that only a small percentage of older Americans have visual impairments or are blind.

Presbyopia, the lack of ability to see objects close to the eyes (farsightedness), usually becomes apparent as one ages, resulting in the need for reading glasses. According to Botwinick (1984), presbyopia actually begins in childhood, but symptoms are usually not noticeable until later in life. The greatest decline in close-distance vision occurs for most people between the ages of 40 and 55 years, and vision declines at a lesser rate thereafter. Schaie and Geiwitz (1982) suggested that most older adults do not experience serious vision problems until they are 80 years or older. They reported that most of the decline in visual abilities of the elderly is attributed to retinal damage, which occurs mainly from faulty blood circulation. Although retinal damage can be seen, according to Schaie and Geiwitz (1982), in most people by the ages of 55 to 65 years, it is usually not debilitating until much later.

Many older people benefit from increased room illumination. This may be because the elderly tend to have smaller eye pupils than younger people, allowing less light to reach the retina. Atchley (1993) reported that the eye of the average 60-year-old person admits only about one-third as much light as the eye of the average 20-year-old person. By raising the level of ambient light, not only acuity but also depth and distance perception may be improved.

A number of ocular problems may afflict older eyes, including cataracts, glaucoma, and macular diseases. Botwinick (1984) estimated that 20 to 25 percent of people in their seventies have cataract problems. With cataracts, the lens of the eye becomes opaque or clouded so that rays of light are scattered in making their way through the visual system. When the condition is advanced, sight may be considerably impaired, and problems with glare may occur. The fact that glare may be uncomfortable may account for why many elderly people prefer a darkened room, rather than a bright, sunny room. Considerable advances have been made in recent years in the surgical treatment of cataracts, either through surgical removal or through implantation of lenses. When the opaque lens has been removed, glare problems should diminish, or even disappear, and sight should be improved.

There is no ideal room illumination for the elderly. Some elderly people may benefit from greater illumination, but a person with cataracts and resultant problems with glare probably does not see well in a highly illuminated space.

Glaucoma, which affects 3 to 5 percent of people older than 65 years (Kline & Schieber, 1985), is a group of eye diseases that involves markedly increased intraocular fluid pressure, changes in the optic nerve, and a reduction of visual field, that is, decreased peripheral vision. Without proper medical treatment, glaucoma can lead to tunnel vision and even to total blindness. Advances have been made in treatment, so substantial loss of visual ability can be avoided by prompt identification.

The color vision of older adults may be distorted. With age, the lenses of the eyes may yellow, thus filtering the shorter wavelengths of light (affecting violet, blue, and green). Colors based on longer wavelengths of light, such as yellows, oranges, and reds are more easily seen. Likewise, age may make it difficult to discriminate the brightness of various colors. Other changes in vision include a narrowing of peripheral vision, reduced secretion of tears, and ocular muscle atrophy.

Hooyman and Kiyak (1988) suggest a number of environmental modifications that help older adults adapt to visual problems. These should be taken into consideration in the design of service delivery settings for the elderly. For example, using high-wattage bulbs, large print on instructional materials, placing contrasting color strips on steps, and reducing glare by installing nonslip and nonglossy floor coverings can reduce the effects of visual disturbances on the elderly. Additional suggestions for modifying both written materials and the physical environment in which audiologic services are provided are given in Chapter 4.

Touch

Another sense that may be affected by age is touch. Deterioration in touch sensitivity in the elderly may be due to changes in the skin and to a loss of nerve endings. Botwinick (1984) reviewed a number of studies that revealed the decline in the sense of touch with age. These studies examined the ability of older adults to manipulate, discriminate, identify, and describe objects based on how they feel. They also delineated striking differences in the use of touch by older and younger people. The ramifications of reduced tactile sensation for manipulation of tiny in-the-canal hearing aids and hearing-aid batteries are addressed in Chapter 3.

Other Senses

The loss of other sensory abilities has been described by gerontologic researchers, including taste, smell, and pain. Because loss of these senses may not have an appreciable impact on an audiologic rehabilitation program, these sensory abilities are not covered herein. The reader is referred to some excellent texts for additional information on these sensory processes— Botwinick (1984); Atchley (1993); Hooyman and Kiyak (1988); Birren & Schaie (1985); Schulz & Ewen (1993).

Financial Changes

According to Atchley (1993), most older people have an adequate income from sources such as employment earnings, assets, and retirement income (Social Security, pensions, and Supplemental Security Income). Since the mid-1970s, there has been a marked increase in the number of older people who have a retirement income in addition to Social Security. In fact, most elderly people now have some form of income beyond Social Security benefits. Atchley reported, however, that a substantial minority of older people has an inadequate income and that the incidence of poverty is much greater among older people than among younger people, especially in minority groups. The trend since the mid-1960s has been for an increasingly more favorable financial outlook for the elderly. Whereas 35.2 percent of older people lived at or below the poverty level in 1959, 14.1 percent of the older population had incomes at or below the poverty level in 1983. Chapter 8 is devoted to a more detailed discussion of financial considerations for audiologists serving the elderly.

Changes in Mobility

One of the changes that may confront older adults and require some changes in lifestyle and activities is mobility. An elderly person may experience a decrease in mobility due to stroke, arthritis, cardiac disorders, or osteoporosis. Additional causes of limited mobility include stiffness of joints, limited visual acuity, and balance problems. As reported by Gioiella and Bevil (1985), however, a radical change in lifestyle is rarely necessary as a result of reduced physical mobility.

Another aspect of mobility in the elderly is transportation. Burrus-Bammel and Bammel (1985) cited a General Accounting Office study in which it was found that 68 percent of elderly people surveyed reported being dependent at least in some degree on others for transportation. The lack, or inconvenience, of transportation to desired activities on the part of elderly people is an obstacle in need of consideration when providing services to this population.

Cognitive Changes

Considerable information has been obtained through formal research on the influence of aging on the three most important cognitive processes: intelligence, memory, and learning. Of these three cognitive processes, intelligence has received the most study and yielded the most controversial results. Hooyman and Kiyak (1988) provide an excellent overview of research in this area. They describe what has been called the *classic aging pattern:* relatively stable performance on the verbal scales of intelligence tests and a worsening with age on the performance subtests of intelligence. The authors noted that the tendency toward poorer performance with age on the performance measures may actually be attributable to age-related changes in certain noncognitive domains, such as sensory, perceptual, and psychomotor abilities. Performance measurements typically tap a person's ability to manipulate familiar and unfamiliar objects, to put a puzzle together, to match a picture, or to arrange pictures in a particular sequence. These tests depend to a greater extent on perceptual and psychomotor skills than do verbal tests, which typically ask for word definitions, social explanations, and descriptions of word and concept similarities. Also, the performance tests on the Wechsler Adult Intelligence Scale (the most widely used measure of adult intelligence) are timed, whereas the verbal tests are not. Botwinick (1984) stated that correlations between chronologic age and intelligence tend to be below .50, often even less than this, thus accounting for only about 25 percent of the variance, at most. Botwinick emphasized that even if higher correlations were evident between intelligence scores and age, these correlations would likely be offset by other characteristics such as wisdom, patience, courage, social adeptness, and a variety of skills not measured during intelligence testing.

Cunningham and Brookbank (1988) observed that most intellectual abilities that are frequently practiced in everyday living situations, such as verbal comprehension and facility with numbers, are not strongly related to age. The implication is that older adults should be expected to perform intellectual tasks as well as they have in the past, if they have reasonably intact health. Kramer (1987) reported that although there is ample evidence in laboratory studies of intellectual decline in later life, the declines are small enough that they would likely have negligible effects on real-life functioning.

Memory, the process of retrieving or recalling information stored in the brain, can be either short-term or long-term. Short-term memory refers to the immediate recall of information, such as repetition of a phone number. Long-term memory involves recall of information hours, days, weeks after absorbing it. According to Poon (1985), research into short-term memory processes has revealed a minimal aging effect. In contrast, striking age effects on long-term memory have been described, and are a source of frustration and embarrassment to older adults. There is evidence, however, that older people can be helped to improve or maintain their long-term memory through techniques such as imagery, mnemonic devices, self-regulation of pace; methods of learning and remembering; organization and elaboration; and practice. Kramer (1987) reported that the content of the memory task has a pronounced effect on older adults' performance. When the material to be remembered, ranging from word lists to prose passages, is familiar or interesting to older adult subjects, age differences disappear, and in some cases older adults outperform younger subjects.

Deterioration in memory in older adults may be due to losses in efficiency of the central nervous system, either as a result of cell death or of less efficient functioning in the areas of the brain that are associated with memory, such as the hippocampus. These changes may be a part of normal aging or due to particular diseases. A number of frequently overlooked causes of memory deterioration in the elderly include medications, depression, and lack of motivation.

Because audiologic rehabilitation of older adults involves learning new information, such as techniques for caring for and using a hearing aid, an understanding of the influence of aging on learning is critical. Hooyman and Kiyak (1988) described a number of factors that may influence learning in the elderly. For example, the physical conditions under which learning takes place, such as lighting, background distractions, comfort, and clarity of the information (either printed or spoken) can have a profound influence on the degree of learning that takes place. The pace of the learning situation also can influence the degree of learning.

The literature on learning by the elderly, as reviewed by Cunningham and Brookbank (1988), suggests that the elderly can and do learn, although learning may be somewhat slow and may require appreciable effort. Botwinick (1984) stated that earlier studies of learning on the part of older adults that showed a pronounced learning deficit may actually have revealed merely a response limitation. In other words, these studies used laboratory tasks that required quick responses, and many of the elderly subjects did not have ample time to demonstrate what they had learned. According to Botwinick (1984), several studies have shown that when adequate response time is allowed, elderly subjects' learning deficits decrease considerably. Cunningham and Brookbank (1988) pointed out that what appears to be a great deal of forgetting by elderly people may actually be poor initial learning. In sum, the literature suggests that the elderly can learn and that their learning may be enhanced by a number of strategies, such as slow presentation of material, repetition and review of materials, and innovative ways to enhance initial learning for better retention.

IMPORTANCE OF COMMUNICATION TO AGING PEOPLE

The importance of communication to the elderly was emphasized by Nussbaum et al (1989). These authors urged that older adults not be viewed as fulfilling a certain prescribed role in society nor as having certain personality profiles but that they be viewed as constantly adapting participants in a system of relationships. These interpersonal relationships are defined by communication behaviors and can have substantial impact on life satisfaction as well as mental and physical health—hence the importance of considering the communication environment of the elderly. Nussbaum et al also noted that communication serves two other important functions for the elderly. First, communication can aid in the loss of mobility that is essential to ensure active participation in family and community. People can maintain at least distant communication with others in the community by using the telephone. Second, communication can aid the elderly in making their special needs known to people who are in a position to help. Williams (1984) emphasized that effective communication is necessary for the elderly to maintain physical independence. Nussbaum et al (1989) cited numerous authors who have developed complex models that predict successful aging. Social interaction is the key determinant of successful aging in each of these models.

The overall communication environment of the elderly must be considered. According to Lubinski (1984), there are two prerequisites for successful communication by older adults: (1) the elderly person must have both the skills and the motivation to communicate, and (2) the external environment of the older person must be conducive to communication. Williams (1984) reported that there are many barriers to effective communication for elderly people in the community. For example, community members may give the impression that they are too busy to talk. Elderly people with hearing impairments are exposed to double jeopardy because of the lack of communication experienced by the elderly combined with the communication problems due to the hearing loss. Exacerbating communication difficulties is the fact that hearing loss is a relatively invisible disorder, and hence community members may react insensitively to any communication breakdowns that may occur. When continued attempts at communication are met with insensitivity, impatience, and intolerance, it is not surprising that many elderly people with hearing impairments retreat from social interaction.

Rather than treat older adults in isolation, the audiologist should determine if a person has likely communication partners. Inclusion of a significant other is one of the most important ingredients for successful rehabilitation of a person with a hearing impairment (see Chapters 5 and 9). The skills of the significant other in communicating with a person with a hearing impairment should be determined. Does the significant other know how to modify his or her message to facilitate comprehension? Does the significant other understand the importance of communication to older adults as well as the frustration that accompanies repeated communication failures? Shadden (1988) recommended that significant others receive information, techniques for management, counseling, support, and a means of sharing.

The ability to communicate, then, is obviously of great importance for maintaining the psychologic and physical independence of the elderly. As audiologists, we have an extremely important role in helping elderly people with hearing impairments to maintain their communication skills. Adequate receptive communication is not a luxury for the aged but is a goal that should be aggressively sought by audiologic practitioners. Lubinski (1984) suggested that speech and hearing professionals who work with older adults view themselves as communication engineers. Efforts must be made to maximize the everyday environment in which communication takes place.

PREVALENCE OF HEARING LOSS IN THE ELDERLY

There have been numerous investigations to document the percentage of the older population with decreased hearing sensitivity. For noninstitutionalized older adults, the percentages vary from 30 percent (Fein, 1983a) to 83 percent (Moscicki et al, 1985). Sommers et al (1982) reported that all of the elderly population in their sample of nursing-home residents demonstrated a hearing impairment. Some of the variation in prevalence can be attributed to the criteria used for defining hearing impairment. For example, using cohorts from the Framingham Heart Study, Moscicki et al (1985) found that 83 percent had hearing impairments, which the authors defined as an elevation of threshold above 20 decibels hearing level (dB HL) in the better ear at any frequency from 250 to 4 kHz. Several years later, Gates et al (1990) used cohorts (60 to 90 years and older) from the Framingham study and found that 29 percent had hearing losses as defined by the criterion of a pure-tone average greater than 26 dB HL in the better ear.

There is general agreement among studies that older men have a higher proportion of hearing problems than older women. In the study by Gates et al (1990), for example, 32.5 percent of men and 26.7 percent of women had a hearing loss.

Because of the aging of the United States population, Fein (1983b) predicted that the percentage of people older than 65 years with hearing impairments will increase to 46 percent by the year 2000 and 59 percent by 2050. The elderly compose the fastest growing segment of American society—the National Center for Health Statistics (1986) determined that hearing impairment is the fourth most prevalent condition affecting the elderly.

Although the estimates of hearing impairments for the older population vary depending on the criteria used for defining hearing loss and the population sampled, there is little debate that as age increases there is a concomitant increase in the incidence of hearing impairment. According to the National Center for Health Statistics (1981, 1982), the rate of hearing impairment increases from 24 percent for people 65 to 74 year of age to 39 percent for people older than 75 years. Dalzell and Puccia (1985) noted that in their young–old group (65 to 69 years of age), the incidence of hearing loss was 56 percent. The incidence increased to 89 percent for the oldest–old group (85 years and older).

AUDIOLOGIC CHARACTERISTICS OF OLDER ADULTS

Age-Related Changes in the Auditory Mechanism

A number of changes occur in the peripheral hearing mechanism as it ages. There is a general loss of elasticity and muscle tonicity throughout the outer ear, including the pinna and the external auditory meatus (Nerbonne, 1988). Earlobes and earlobe creases appear to grow with age. The skin in the external canal shows atrophy and thinning; manipulation may cause it to crack and bleed. There is a decrease in cerumen production, concomitant with atrophy and decreased activity of the glands (White & Regan, 1987). In the middle ear, the tympanic membrane stiffens. The fibers of the tensor tympani and stapedius muscles lose their elasticity. There is also progressive degeneration of the incudomalleal and incudostapedial joints of the ossicles due to arthritis. These middle ear changes seem to have minimal effects on hearing (Maurer & Rupp, 1979; White & Regan, 1987).

Age-related changes also occur in the inner ear. These changes are much more detrimental to the hearing sensitivity of the person. Inner ear changes were first observed and described by Schuknecht in 1955; the observations were made during postmortem histopathologic studies and audiometric testing. Schuknecht observed atrophic changes in the membranous labyrinth and in the efferent and afferent fibers of the organ of Corti. He also described degenerative changes and a decrease in the number of auditory neurons. Schuknecht called these changes *presbycusis*, which he classified into four age-related patterns (Schuknecht, 1974). Sensory presbycusis is characterized by hair cell loss in the basal end of the cochlea, neural degeneration, atrophy of the organ of Corti, and high-frequency hearing loss. Strial presbycusis is characterized by atrophy of the stria vascularis, which results in a decreased supply of nutrition to the cochlea. There is little hair cell loss and the audiometric pattern is flat. Neural presbycusis is characterized by degeneration of the cochlear neurons rather than the sensory elements. This loss of neurons is also present in the central nervous system. These patients demonstrate phonemic regression or speech discrimination disproportionately poorer than predicted by a pure-tone audiogram. Cochlear conductive presbycusis is characterized by stiffening of the basilar membrane and atrophy of the spiral ligament (Schuknecht, 1974).

Two other types of presbycusis were identified by Johnsson and Hawkins (1979). These are vascular presbycusis, which is characterized by a loss of the minute blood vessels that supply the stria vascularis, spiral ligament, and tympanic lip, and central presbycusis, characterized by a loss of neurons from the cochlear nucleus and other auditory centers of the brain. The six types of presbycusis rarely occur separately.

The degeneration and atrophy described in presbycusis are not limited to the peripheral system. There appears to be a degeneration of some cells, a decrease in the number of neurons, and an increase in the accumulation of pigment in other cells throughout the central auditory mechanism in aged adults (Feldman & Vaughan, 1979). A decrease in the ability to perceive the complex impulses of speech may be related to this loss of healthy cells.

Gates et al (1990) described three major etiologic factors associated with hearing losses in the elderly: intrinsic, age-related degeneration; noise damage from recreational, occupational, and everyday exposure; and biologic effects of diseases, ototoxic agents, and diet, superimposed on a genetic mechanism. Thus, presbycusis is not a simple matter of degeneration of the auditory mechanism due to age, but a complex phenomenon possibly encompassing the interaction of several etiologic factors, which are more likely to occur with advancing age.

Audiologic Findings in Older Adults

Presbycusis is most commonly characterized by a gradually sloping, high-frequency loss that is typically bilateral and symmetric. It has been well documented that the loss begins gradually and accelerates with advancing age. In addition to the decrease in pure-tone sensitivity, it is generally assumed that the ability to understand speech diminishes as age increases. Gaeth (1948) was the first to observe this phenomenon. He noted a disproportionate loss in speech discrimination in patients with hearing impairments who were older than 60 years. A number of investigators have reported that elderly people tend to do more poorly on speech discrimination tests than do younger subjects (Jerger, 1973; Bess & Townsend, 1977). Other investigators (Surr, 1977) have found no statistically significant differences between young and elderly adults in speech discrimination when audiograms are matched between the two age groups. In the study by Gates et al (1990), only 0.3 percent of the Framingham Heart Study cohorts had disproportionately poor word recognition scores.

Although there is a degree of uncertainty as to the effect of aging on the ability to discriminate speech in quiet environments, the older population generally experiences more difficulty when speech is degraded (Schow et al, 1978). A common description by older adults is, "I hear fine in quiet situations but I have difficulty when there are several people talking at once or when it is noisy."

The decreased performance of the elderly on speech tasks that have been altered or degraded has been well documented and supports what Jerger and Hayes (1977) call central aging effects. That is, in addition to the peripheral impairment associated with aging, the higher auditory pathways may be involved. In one study by Hayes and Jerger, 18 percent of the subjects were classified as having central impairments (Hayes & Jerger, 1979a), whereas in another, 42 percent had central involvement (Hayes & Jerger, 1979b). Shirinian and Arnst (1982) reported an incidence of 74 percent for central auditory involvement, whereas Kricos et al (1987) found that 58 percent of their older patients had a central component to their hearing losses. Stach et al (1990) found a pronounced effect of age on the incidence of central presbycusis; there was a prevalence of 95 percent in the age group 80 years and older.

Study of the nature of speech understanding difficulties among the elderly is difficult because of the complexity of the speech perception process and the number of variables that must be controlled, such as age, cognitive status, and degree of hearing loss. Humes and Christopherson (1991) found that elevated thresholds in the elderly account for most of their speech identification difficulties. Another factor found, although not as pronounced as degree of hearing loss, was auditory processing ability, that is, the ability to discriminate acoustic stimuli on the basis of parameters such as intensity, frequency, and duration. Humes (1991), Humes et al (1994), and Souza and Turner (1994) argue that loss of hearing sensitivity plays an important role in the speech recognition difficulties of the elderly. Jerger (1992), however, in a study carefully constructed to control for degree of hearing sensitivity, found an age-related decline in synthetic sentence identification that could not be satisfactorily explained by peripheral hearing loss or by cognitive status. Similarly, Gordon-Salant and Fitzgibbons (1993) concluded that age-related factors other than peripheral hearing loss contribute to the speech recognition difficulties of the elderly. Jerger et al (1994) showed that aging causes a progressive decline in the central processing of speech and that the decline is more pronounced for left-ear input than for right-ear input. These authors demonstrated that the ear effects were not due to differences in hearing sensitivity between the ears.

Crandell et al (1991) noted that elderly listeners with similar audiograms may vary considerably in their abilities to recognize speech in adverse listening environments and that the physiologic origins of these speech recognition difficulties remain uncertain. Their review of the literature regarding speech perception in the aged revealed three main hypotheses for the origin of speech recognition difficulties: cochlear, central, or cognitive dysfunction. Crandell et al suggested that for many elderly listeners, problems with speech recognition result from the complex interaction of peripheral hearing loss, central pathway deterioration, and cognitive dysfunction.

Implications of Hearing Loss for the Older Adult

Hearing loss has both direct and indirect influences on the quality of life for older adults. The direct consequences are a reduction of speech perception performance in quiet and noisy situations. The indirect consequences may include psychologic repercussions that reduce a person's ability to make full use of available sensory input channels to learn new skills or to sustain the motivation for interpersonal communication. Depression, embarrassment, frustration, social isolation, anger, and fear are often caused by an elderly person's inability to communicate because of a hearing loss.

A hearing impairment may inhibit a person's ability to function independently. It may affect quality of life and cause safety problems. Interactions with family and friends may suffer. Because of increasing difficulties with communication, elderly people with hearing impairments may isolate themselves from family, friends, and previously enjoyed social activities. Older adults with hearing impairment may not want to attend religious services, the theater, or group activities. They may not want to listen to the radio or watch television. They may find it difficult to communicate with physicians and tradespeople. Lack of ability to hear people and vehicles approaching, pots boiling, alarm systems, the telephone, doorbell, and television or radio emergency announcements are some of the safety hazards.

The effects of hearing loss are apparent regardless of whether a person with a hearing impairment is young or old. Given the severe difficulties many elderly people experience with speech perception in adverse listening environments, elderly people with hearing impairments are at an even greater risk for communication difficulties and subsequent psychosocial ramifications than are young people. Gordon-Salant et al (1994) found that younger people with hearing losses reported more handicapping effects than elderly people with hearing losses. The authors suggested that this finding might be due to the greater communication demands faced by younger people or to the gradual progression of hearing loss in the elderly. The findings highlight the need for helping the elderly to understand the impact of hearing loss on communication.

CONCLUSION

The physical, sensory, and lifestyle changes experienced by the elderly must be addressed in the design of effective and relevant audiologic rehabilitation programs for this population.

REFERENCES

Atchley, R.C. (1993). *The social forces and aging: An introduction to social gerontology*. Belmont: Wadsworth.

Bess, F.H., & Townsend, T.H. (1977). Word discrimination for listeners with flat sensorineural hearing losses. *Journal of Speech and Hearing Disorders, 42,* 232-237.

Birren, J.E., & Schaie, K.W. (1985). *Handbook of the psychology of aging*. New York: Van Nostrand Reinhold.

Botwinick, J. (1984). *Aging and behavior.* New York: Springer Publishing.

Burrus-Bammel, L.L., & Bammel, G. (1985). Leisure and recreation. In J.E. Birren & F. Schieber (Eds.), *Handbook of the psychology of aging* (pp. 848-864). New York: Van Nostrand Reinhold.

Cox, H.G. (1988). *Later life: The realities of aging.* Englewood Cliffs: Prentice Hall.

Crandell, C.C., Henoch, M.A., & Dunkerson, K.A. (1991). A review of speech perception and aging: Some implications for aural rehabilitation. *Journal of the Academy of Rehabilitative Audiology, 24,* 121-132.

Cunningham, W.R., & Brookbank, J.W. (1988). *Gerontology: The psychology, biology, and sociology of aging.* New York: Harper & Row.

Dalzell, L.E., & Puccia, D.S. (1985). Hearing loss and hearing handicap in the oldest–old. Presented at the Annual Convention of the American Speech-Language-Hearing Association, November 22-25, 1985, Washington, D.C.

Fein, D.J. (1983a). The prevalence of speech and language impairments. *ASHA, 25,* 37.

Fein, D.J. (1983b). Projections of speech and hearing impairments to 2050. *ASHA, 25,* 31.

Feldman, M.L., & Vaughan, D.W. (1979). Changes in the auditory pathway with age. In S.S. Han & D.H. Coons (Eds.), *Special senses in aging: A current biological assessment* (pp. 143-162). Ann Arbor: Institute of Gerontology, University of Michigan.

Gaeth, J. (1948). *A study of phonemic regression in relation to hearing loss.* Evanston: Northwestern University. Dissertation.

Gates, G.A., Cooper, J.C., Kannel, W.B., & Miller, N.J. (1990). Hearing in the elderly: The Framingham Cohort, 1983–1985. I. Basic audiometric test results. *Ear and Hearing, 11,* 247-256.

Gioiella, E.C., & Bevil, C.W. (1985). *Nursing care of the aging client: Promoting healthy adaptation.* Norwalk: Appleton-Century-Crofts.

Gordon-Salant, S., & Fitzgibbons, P.J. (1993). Temporal factors and speech recognition performance in young and elderly listeners. *Journal of Speech and Hearing Research, 36,* 1276-1285.

Hayes, D., & Jerger, J. (1979a). Aging and the use of hearing aids. *Scandinavian Audiology, 8,* 33-40.

Hayes, D., & Jerger, J. (1979b). Low-frequency hearing loss in presbycusis: A central interpretation. *Archives of Otolaryngology, 105,* 9-12.

Hendricks, J., & Hendricks, C.D. (1986). *Aging in mass society: Myths & realities.* Boston: Little, Brown.

Hooyman, N.R., & Kiyak, H. A. (1988). *Social gerontology: A multidisciplinary perspective.* Boston: Allyn & Bacon.

Humes, L.E. (1991). Understanding the speech understanding problems of the hearing impaired. *Journal of the American Academy of Audiology, 2,* 59-69.

Humes, L.E., & Christopherson, L. (1991). Speech identification difficulties of hearing-impaired elderly persons: The contributions of auditory processing deficits. *Journal of Speech and Hearing Research, 34,* 686-693.

Humes L.E., Watson B.U., Christensen L.A., Cokely C.G., Halling D.C., & Lee L. (1994). Factors associated with individual differences in clinical measures of speech recognition among the elderly. *Journal of Speech and Hearing Research, 37,* 465-474.

Jerger, J. (1973). Audiological findings in aging. *Advances in Oto-Rhino-Laryngology, 20,* 115-124.

Jerger, J. (1992) Can age-related decline in speech understanding be explained by peripheral hearing loss? *Journal of the American Academy of Audiology, 3,* 33-38.

Jerger J., Chmiel R., Allen J., & Wilson A. (1994). Effects of age and gender on dichotic sentence identification. *Ear and Hearing, 15,* 274-286.

Jerger, J., & Hayes, D. (1977). Diagnostic speech audiometry. *Archives of Otolaryngology, 102,* 216-222.

Johnsson, L.G., & Hawkins, J.E. (1979). Age-related degeneration of the inner ear. In S.S. Han & D.H. Coons (Eds.), *Special senses in aging: A current biological assessment* (pp. 119-135). Ann Arbor: Institute of Gerontology, University of Michigan.

Kart, C.S. (1994). *The realities of aging: An introduction to gerontology.* Boston: Allyn & Bacon.

Kline, D.W., & Schieber, F. (1985). Vision and aging. In J.E. Birren & F. Schieber (Eds.), *Handbook of the psychology of aging* (pp. 296-331). New York: Van Nostrand Reinhold.

Korper, S.P. (1989). Epidemiologic and demographic characteristics of the aging population. In J.G. Goldstein, H.K. Kushimu, & C.F. Koopmann (Eds.), *Geriatric otorhinolaryngology* (pp. 19-29). Toronto: Decker.

Kramer, D.A. (1987). Cognition and aging: The emergence of a new tradition. In P. Silverman (Ed.), *The elderly as modern pioneers.* Bloomington: Indiana University Press.

Kricos, P.B., Lesner, S.A., Sandridge, S.A., & Yanke, R.L. (1987). Perceived benefits of amplification as a function of central auditory status in the elderly. *Ear and Hearing, 8,* 337-342.

Lubinski, R. (1984) The environmental role in communication skills and opportunities of older people. In C. Wilder & B. Weinstein (Eds.), *Aging and communication: Problems in management.* New York: Haworth.

Maurer, J.F., & Rupp, R.R. (1979). The aging auditory process. In J.F. Maurer & R.R. Rupp (Eds.), *Hearing and aging* (pp. 36-66). New York: Grune & Stratton.

Moscicki, E.K., Elkins, E.F., Baum, H.M., & McNamara, P.M. (1985). Hearing loss in the elderly: An epidemiologic study of the Framingham Heart Study cohort. *Ear and Hearing, 6,* 184-190.

National Center for Health Statistics (1981). Prevalence of selected impairments: United States 1977. *Vital and health statistics.* DHHS Publication No. 81-1562. Washington: United States Government Printing Office.

National Center for Health Statistics (1982). Hearing ability of persons by sociodemographic and health characteristics: United States. *Vital and health statistics.* DHHS Publication No. 82-1568. Washington: United States Government Printing Office.

National Center for Health Statistics (1986). Prevalence of selected chronic conditions: United States 1979–1981. *Vital and health statistics.* Series 10, No. 155. DHHS Publication. No. (PHS) 86-1583. Washington, D.C.: United States Government Printing Office.

Nerbonne, M.A. (1988). The effects of aging on auditory structures and functions. In B.B. Shadden (Ed.), *Communication behavior and aging: A source book for clinicians* (pp. 137-161). Baltimore: Williams & Wilkins.

Neugarten, B.L. (1975). The future and the young–old. *The Gerontologist, 15,* 4-9.

Nussbaum, J.F., Thompson, T., & Robinson, J.D. (1989). *Communication and aging.* New York: Harper & Row.

Piscopo, J. (1985). Physical health and wellness of older adults. In T. Tedrick (Ed.), *Aging: Issues and policies for the 1980's* (pp. 50-61). New York: Praeger.

Poon, L.W. (1985). Differences in human memory with aging: Nature, causes, and clinical implications. In J.E. Birren and K.W. Schaie (Eds.), *Handbook of the psychology of aging* (2nd ed.) (pp. 427-462). New York: Van Nostrand Reinhold.

Schaie, K.W., & Geiwitz, J. (1982). *Adult development and aging.* Boston: Little, Brown.

Schow, R.L., Christensen, J.M., Hutchinson, J.M., & Nerbonne, M.A. (1978). *Communication disorders of the aged.* Baltimore: University Park Press.

Schuknecht, H.F. (1955). Presbycusis. *Laryngoscope, 65,* 402-419.

Schuknecht, H.F. (1974). *Pathology of the ear.* Cambridge: Harvard University Press.

Schulz, R., & Ewen, R.B. (1993). Adult development and aging. New York: Macmillan.

Shadden, B.B. (1988). Education, counseling, and support for significant others. In B.B. Shadden (Ed.), *Communication behavior and aging: A sourcebook for clinicians* (pp. 309-329). Baltimore: Williams & Wilkins.

Shanas, E. (1980). Social myth as hypothesis: The case of the family relations of old people. In G.L. Landreth & R.C. Berg (Eds.), *Counseling the elderly: For professional helpers who work with the aged.* Springfield: Thomas.

Shirinian, M.J., & Arnst, D.J. (1982). Patterns in the performance-intensity functions for phonetically balanced word lists and synthetic sentences in aged listeners. *Archives of Otolaryngology, 108,* 15-20.

Silverman, P. (1987). Introduction: The life course perspective. In P. Silverman (Ed.), *The elderly as modern pioneers.* Bloomington: Indiana University Press.

Sommers, R.K., Weidner, W.E., & McAleer, C. (1982). Audiometric threshold levels of nursing home residents. *Hearing Aid Journal, 35,* 19-21.

Souza P.E., & Turner C.W. (1994). Masking of speech in young and elderly listeners with hearing loss. *Journal of Speech and Hearing Research, 37,* 665-661.

Stach, B.A., Spretnjak, M.L., & Jerger, J. (1990). The prevalence of central presbycusis in a clinical population. *Journal of the American Academy of Audiology, 1,* 109-115.

Surr, R. (1977). Effect of age on clinic hearing aid evaluation results. *Journal of the American Auditory Society, 3,* 1-5.z

White, J.D., & Regan, M.M.S. (1987). Otologic considerations. In H.G. Mueller & V.C. Geoffrey (Eds.), *Communication disorders in aging: Assessment and management* (pp. 36-71). Washington: Gallaudet University Press.

Williams, P.S. (1984). *Hearing loss: Information for professionals in the aging network.* Washington: National Information Center on Deafness, Gallaudet College.

Chapter 2

Audiologic Rehabilitation Assessment: A Holistic Approach

Sharon A. Lesner and Patricia B. Kricos

Assessment is an important first step in the audiologic rehabilitation process. The purpose of assessment should be to gain an understanding of how a patient functions, including the patient's abilities, limitations, and perceived needs. On the basis of the findings an audiologic rehabilitation treatment plan can be tailored for the patient and the patient's family or significant other persons (SOPs). Results of the assessment may provide a baseline for pre- and postintervention comparisons and may signal the need for referrals for other professional services.

To be effective, audiologic rehabilitation assessment should be holistic and should include both formal and informal measures. The sum is greater than the parts, and to understand function, one must consider the interrelations of several factors. In addition to communication ability, interactions among the patient's physical, psychologic, and social status contribute to the manner in which the person functions (Figure 2–1).

In addition, although portions of the assessment can take place in the clinical environment, it is desirable for evaluations to be made in the actual environments in which the patient functions. Ecologic assessments are gaining in popularity in vision care, and they seem particularly suited for hearing care (Hiatt, 1990). If time and cost preclude an ecologic assessment, simulated environments should be used. For example, if a patient is having difficulty hearing in a reverberant room, the reverberation time can be recreated electronically in the clinic.

Audiologic rehabilitation assessment must extend beyond audiologic assessment if intervention is to be optimized. Although it is important to know about the status of the person's hearing, it is even more important in the development of a treatment plan to know about the person who has the hearing loss. In fact, a guiding principle should be to determine the strengths, capabilities, and needs of the person with the hearing impairment and not focus only on the person's hearing status. This is especially so considering that older adults may have several chronic health problems as well as age-appropriate biologic and psychologic changes that must be considered (Hartke,

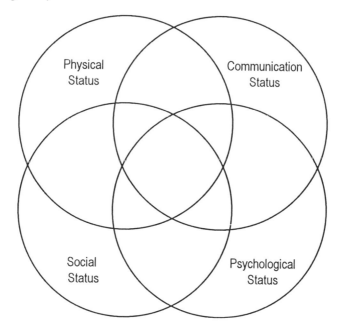

FIGURE 2–1   *Domains for assessment.*

1991). With the variety of factors that affect function, no single battery of tests fits all patients or all situations.

Although several assessment domains exist, the practitioner must keep in mind that assessments do not help the patient. It is the outcome of assessments that lead to actions that may help patients (Kane, 1990). Over-evaluation, especially during the first few sessions, should be avoided. Otherwise, patients may perceive that the practitioner is more interested in testing than in providing care. The purpose of this chapter is to highlight the components of audiologic rehabilitation assessment that can assist in the development of effective hearing care for older adults. The components shown in Table 2–1 and Appendix 2–1 are emphasized.

TABLE 2–1   Global Assessment Domains for Audiologic Rehabilitation

PHYSICAL STATUS
General health
Visual status (acuity, ocular disease)
Dexterity and fine motor skills (proximal, distal)

PSYCHOLOGIC STATUS
Mental status
Motivation
Attitude
Depression

TABLE 2–1 Global Assessment Domains for Audiologic Rehabilitation (continued)

SOCIOLOGIC STATUS
Social environment

Physical environment

COMMUNICATION STATUS
Hearing handicap or disability

Auditory speech reception

Speechreading

Audiovisual speech reception

Conversational fluency

GLOBAL ASSESSMENT DOMAINS

Physical Status

General Health

General health status contributes to the amount of interest in, strength for, and motivation for audiologic rehabilitation. A large percentage of people older than 65 years have chronic illnesses. The most common chronic health problems experienced by people older than 65 years are listed in Table 2–2. Preoccupation with an illness generally takes precedence over hearing problems, because hearing problems do not typically represent a crisis. Health problems may necessitate modification of the environment in which treatment is provided (eg, orthopedic or visual problems) and in the scheduling of sessions (eg, incontinence or fatigue). Several potential side effects of drug use, such as nervousness, confusion, and lethargy, may affect treatment. Health status and the use of medications should be explored during history-taking. Problems must then be anticipated and accounted for.

TABLE 2–2 Most Common Chronic Conditions Among People 65 Years or Older

Condition	Cases per 1000 Population
Arthritis	482.2
Heart disease	442.9
Hypertension	371.1
Hearing loss	296.8
Orthopedic problem	165.3
Cataracts	161.7
Chronic sinusitis	145.3
Diabetes	98.2

TABLE 2–2　Most Common Chronic Conditions Among People 65 Years or Older
(continued)

Condition	Cases per 1000 Population
Tinnitus	85.5
Vision impairment	77.4

(Reprinted from National Center for Health Statistics 1987)

Visual Status

Vision impairment is common among older adults. The prevalence is more than 46 percent among people older than 85 years (Roth, 1991). The most common problems are discussed in Chapter 1. Vision is important for speechreading. Acuity of 20/40 is needed for optimal performance (Hardick et al, 1970). Adequate vision is needed for manipulation of hearing aids, use of assistive devices, and for audiologic rehabilitation programming. Patients should be asked about their vision status, and vision screenings with a device such as a Jaeger card or Snellen chart or Titmus, Keystone, or Ortho-Rater vision tester, should be routine. (We know of one patient who was functionally blind yet received 10 weeks of speechreading therapy.) The results of the screening can alert the audiologist to the need for referrals or for the need to alter treatment (Herkind et al, 1983).

Dexterity and Fine Motor Skills

Successful manipulation of hearing aids and batteries requires the user to have both proximal and distal arm function. Proximal function involves the ability to raise the arms, and distal function involves manual dexterity (Lachs et al, 1990). Several pathologic processes, especially arthritis, may cause functional disability. A patient's ability to manipulate hearing aids, batteries, and assistive listening devices should be routinely assessed with direct observation. Although it is important to assure that a patient can manage a prosthetic device at the time of dispensing, it is also critical that retention of the skills be reassessed during the trial period. Many older adults experience short-term memory problems and may consequently forget how to insert hearing aids or use assistive listening devices. Older adults often have reduced pain sensitivity. It is not uncommon for a hearing-aid wearer to have a sore ear because of a poorly fitting earmold and not be aware of the problem.

If difficulties exist, changes in the style or size of the devices, batteries, or accessories may be needed. If a patient cannot handle a hearing aid, the audiologist should consider the use of assistive devices. When problems exist, a SOP should be identified and provided with counseling about the hearing loss and the use of the hearing aids or assistive listening devices. Inclusion of a SOP in group audiologic rehabilitation is absolutely necessary (see Chapter 9). Audiologists should also consider referring the patient to an occupational or physical therapist.

Psychologic Status

Mental Status

Careful observation of patients provides an opportunity to evaluate their appearance and behavior. Affect, orientation, memory, judgment, and perception should be observed and documented (Cadieux et al, 1985). Observation alone, however, is not sufficient to identify cognitive disorders among older adults. As many as 10 percent of people older than 65 years have mild to moderate cognitive impairment sufficient to affect performance of everyday activities (Gallo et al, 1988; LaFerle & LaFerle, 1988). Older people often compensate for the presence of cognitive impairment, and some patients with borderline normal mental status may appear to function well because of the help provided by a SOP. Therefore, screening of mental status should be routine (Lachs et al, 1990).

If a cognitive impairment is identified, the patient should still be considered a candidate for audiologic rehabilitation. However, it is important in these cases to enlist the help of a SOP.

Although there are several validated screening tests for mental status, loss of short-term memory and calculation ability tend to be sensitive indicators of cognitive impairment (Lachs et al, 1990). We have found that the Short Portable Mental Status Questionnaire (Pfeiffer, 1975) and the Folstein Mini Mental State (Folstein et al, 1975) are excellent screening tools. When the mental status tests are administered, patients are told that they will be asked some questions that may seem rather strange but that the questions are routinely asked of all patients.

Motivation

According to Kemp (1990), motivation is one of the most important factors that determine rehabilitative success. Motivation is what a patient wants to or does not want to do. For example, a practitioner may believe a patient who refuses to wear a hearing aid has low motivation. The person may be receiving extra help and special attention from a SOP because of the inability to hear. If the patient wants the special attention, then the patient will be motivated to maintain the status quo.

Kemp (1990) suggested that motivation can be evaluated by determining what a patient really wants, what he or she believes will occur if the goal is to be achieved, and what rewards are likely to occur. All of these factors are influenced by the physical, economic, emotional, and social costs. The relationship between these components is shown in the following equation:

$$\text{Motivation} = \frac{\text{Wants} \times \text{Beliefs} \times \text{Rewards}}{\text{Costs}}$$

Certain age-related changes may make older people appear to be less motivated than younger patients. Factors include a tendency toward the status quo, avoidance of risk taking, needing more time to make decisions, and the avoidance of failure (Kemp, 1986). An understanding of a person's motivation requires that the audiologist establish a helping and open relationship and then help determine wants, beliefs, rewards, and costs. Information should be obtained from the patient and the SOP.

Attitude

A person's attitude toward his or her hearing and toward potential rehabilitation is the key to the outcome. Goldstein and Stephens (1981) suggested that candidates for audiologic rehabilitation fall within one of the four attitude types (Table 2–3 (Goldstein & Stephens, 1981)). Approximately two-thirds to three-fourths of patients seen in an audiology clinic are Type I, and most of the rest are Type II. Type can be determined from the patient's history and with interviews of both the patient and the SOP.

Even patients who are essentially negative or strongly negative are candidates for audiologic rehabilitation, especially if group audiologic rehabilitation is provided and the patient is assisted in working through the denial. It is important for the audiologist to show a great deal of patience (Piercy & Goldstein, 1994).

Depression

Depression occurs frequently among older adults; it is an important factor in the determination of rehabilitative potential (Trezona, 1991). For community

---

TABLE 2–3   Types of Patients Who Seek Audiologic Rehabilitation

TYPE I. STRONG POSITIVE

The patient has a strong positive attitude toward hearing aids and audiologic rehabilitation. The patient has realistic expectations and both understands and accepts the problem. No other complicating factors exist.

TYPE II. POSITIVE

The patient is positive about hearing aids and rehabilitation, but some complication exists. Audiometric configuration, special needs, psychologic or social variables may make treatment more involved than would otherwise be true.

TYPE III. ESSENTIALLY NEGATIVE

The patient has a negative attitude—expressed or unexpressed—toward the hearing aid or therapy.

TYPE IV. STRONG NEGATIVE

The patient rejects hearing aids and audiologic rehabilitation. Even if treatment would be beneficial, the patient denies the existence of a problem.

residents, the prevalence of depression is 13 to 15 percent; among disabled older adults, the prevalence rises to 20 to 30 percent (Blazer & Williams, 1980). It is important to remember that depression is not normal at any age (Morgan, 1989).

Depression causes a loss of energy, and the patient loses interest in receiving rehabilitative services. Depressed patients can have a negative effect on group work because of impaired memory and concentration. In addition, the irritability and sense of hopelessness associated with depression can serve to alienate other patients and the professional staff (Trezona, 1991). Depression is one of the most frequently occurring conditions associated with suicide among the elderly (Richman, 1991).

Several instruments and scales are available to measure depression (Gallo et al, 1988). Lachs et al (1990) suggested that use of the single simple question "Do you often feel sad or depressed?" can serve as a simple screening device. People who respond in the affirmative can be administered a formal scale such as the Geriatric Depression Scale (Yesavage & Brink, 1983). More important, because of the possibility of suicide, appropriate referrals should be made.

Social Status

The environment within which a patient functions must be assessed. The communication environment includes both physical and social environments. The physical environment includes the spaces a person inhabits, and the social environment consists of the people with whom a person lives and regularly interacts (Hiatt, 1990). Both physical and social environments should be evaluated within an ecologic framework so that appropriate environmental, instrumental, or behavioral care can be provided and then evaluated for effectiveness.

Lubinski (1984) suggested that there are two prerequisites for successful communication by older adults: (1) the elderly person must have both the skills and the motivation to communicate, and (2) the external environment of the older person must be conducive to communication. A goal of the audiologist should be to modify the environment so that it is as safe and accessible as possible and so that communication is optimized.

Social Environment

The audiologist must determine with whom the patient frequently communicates and with whom the patient experiences the greatest communication difficulties. If possible, those people should be included in the audiologic rehabilitation treatment plan. SOPs should receive information, techniques for management, counseling, support, and a means of sharing (Shadden, 1988).

Physical Environment

The patient should be asked about where they experience communication problems. The nature of the communication problems experienced at home, places of worship, and in recreational, vocational, educational, and social settings should be determined so that appropriate recommendations can be provided. A visit to the various sites by the audiologist assists in determining the need for modifications of ambient noise, behavioral modifications, or use of assistive listening devices or special hearing-aid circuits, programs, or features. If assistive listening devices or special hearing-aid fittings are needed, the audiologist should demonstrate the use of and benefit of the devices in the actual setting in which they will be used. If that is not possible, simulated environments should be used.

ASSESSMENT OF HEARING HANDICAP

Self-assessment scales or inventories provide an effective method for the systematic assessment of the emotional and social consequences of hearing impairment for the patient as well as SOPs. The primary purposes of these scales are to determine whether a hearing impairment has manifested itself as a hearing handicap and to quantify the amount of the handicap. As shown in Chapter 1, there is only a moderate correlation between audiometric results and self-perceived handicap. Knowing that an older adult has a 45 decibel hearing level (dB HL) hearing loss provides little insight to the audiologist about whether the person's social, emotional, vocational, and communication well-being are affected by the hearing loss. As Ross (1987) showed, the use of self-assessment scales is necessary to define the rehabilitative needs of our patients.

A number of self-report assessment scales have been developed. The basic format of these instruments consists of presenting the person with the hearing impairment with a series of questions relating to potentially handicapping situations or conditions and asking the person to judge his or her overall performance, attitude, and perception in terms of the effects of the hearing loss on the examples given in the inventory. Some of the hearing handicap scales are relatively short, such as the Hearing Handicap Inventory for the Elderly—Screening Version (Ventry & Weinstein, 1983) and the Self-Assessment of Communication (Schow & Nerbonne, 1982), both of which contain ten items. These brief inventories can be used to screen older adults to determine whether hearing loss is perceived to be a handicap (ASHA Report, 1992). This information, in turn, can be used to determine who may be candidates for hearing aids, assistive devices, and audiologic rehabilitation. Longer scales, such as the 90-item Hearing Performance Inventory (Giolas et al, 1979) and the 145-item Communication Profile for the Hearing

Impaired (Demorest & Erdman, 1986; 1987), may provide more detailed information about the psychosocial effects of the hearing loss.

In addition to providing information to the audiologist, the administration of a handicap scale may be therapeutic in itself. The actual process of self-reflection that the older adult undergoes as the inventory is completed may lead to insights into the problems experienced and the person's reactions (both positive and negative) to them. Giolas et al (1979) suggested that audiologists may use inventory items as starting points for discussion during counseling with adults with hearing impairments.

McCarthy et al (1990) described three potential uses of hearing handicap inventories. One application would be in counseling. Several handicap scales have versions for both the person with the hearing impairment and their SOPs (eg, spouse, family members, nursing home staff). These allow a comparison between the patient's perception of hearing handicap and that of the SOP. They also enable the audiologist to gather important information regarding the attitudes and perceptions of family members to be used during counseling.

A second use of hearing handicap inventories, according to McCarthy et al (1990), is to determine the benefit of a hearing aid. Because one of the primary goals of hearing-aid fitting is to reduce the communication and psychosocial handicaps associated with hearing loss, a hearing handicap inventory may provide information about whether the goal has been met. Several authors have reported the use of hearing handicap inventories to document the benefits of hearing-aid use (Malinoff & Weinstein, 1989a, 1989b; Newman & Weinstein, 1988).

McCarthy et al (1990) suggested that handicap inventories may be useful for quality assurance. As insurance carriers continue to require increasingly specific documentation and care plans, self-assessment inventories may provide useful information for admission and discharge criteria. These inventories also may provide measurements of treatment outcomes, effectiveness, and quality.

A review of the handicap inventories that seem most relevant for assessment of older adults with hearing impairments is presented herein. The two we use most frequently with our elderly clients, The Hearing Handicap Inventory for the Elderly (HHIE) (Ventry & Weinstein, 1982) and the Self-Assessment of Communication (SAC) (Schow & Nerbonne, 1982) are reproduced in Appendixes 2–2 and 2–3. We use these instruments most frequently because they have undergone standardization and their brevity. is attractive in a busy audiology practice. In choosing which scale to use, the practitioner is faced with the dilemma of picking a scale, such as the HHIE or SAC, that provides general perception of hearing handicap in a matter of minutes, or choosing a longer instrument such as the Communication Profile for the Hearing Impaired (CPHI) (Demorest & Erdman, 1986; 1987), which provides detailed information but would likely be unpractical for an audiologist who treats many patients.

Palmer (1992) discussed the possibilities of computer administration and scoring of hearing performance inventories, which would be particularly helpful for the longer inventories such as the CPHI. Potential problems with computer administration include the unfamiliarity of many adults, perhaps especially older adults, with computer keyboards and mouse pads, which might influence results; glare from a computer monitor; loss of human interaction; and lack of standardization of computer-administered inventories. A database system for scoring the CPHI is available from CPHI Services, PO Box 444, Simpsonville, MD 21150-0444. Scoring programs for the HPI, HHIE, and the Performance Inventory for Profound and Severe Loss (PIPSL) (Owens & Raggio, 1988) can be obtained from the Support Syndicate for Audiology, 108 South 12th Street, Pittsburgh, PA 15203, telephone 800-869-0758.

Hearing Handicap Scales

The Denver Scale of Communication Function

The Denver Scale of Communication Function (Alpiner et al, unpublished study, 1974) focuses on the attitudes and feelings of people with hearing impairments and their SOPs. The scale consists of 25 statements rated on a seven-point scale between "agree" and "disagree." The statements cover four areas: family, self, social-vocational, and general communication experiences. A profile chart in the scoring section specifies the strengths and weaknesses of the person with the hearing impairment.

Hearing Performance Inventory

The Hearing Performance Inventory (HPI) (Giolas et al, 1979) was developed to assess hearing performance in problem areas of communication in everyday listening situations. Inventory items are divided into six categories: understanding speech, intensity, response to auditory failure, social, personal, and occupational. The person being tested is presented with everyday listening situations and asked to evaluate the frequency with which they experience a particular degree of performance—most often degree of difficulty (practically always, frequently, about half the time, occasionally, and almost never). The HPI has 90 items, 15 of which are concerned with occupational situations, which may be omitted for elderly who are not employed.

The Hearing Handicap Inventory for the Elderly

The HHIE (Ventry & Weinstein, 1982) was designed to assess the effects of hearing impairment on the emotional and social adjustment of elderly people who do not live in institutions. The inventory comprises two subscales: a 13-item subscale explores the emotional consequences of hearing impairment, and a 12-item subscale explores both social and situational effects. The HHIE was standardized on the basis of results for people older than 60 years. It has been shown to be a reliable and valid method for identifying handicapping hearing impairments among older adults (Lichtenstein et al, 1988; Weinstein, 1986). The sensitivity and specificity rates of the HHIE are 70 to 80 percent for identifying hearing losses of moderate or greater degree (American Academy of Audiology, 1991). A screening version (HHIE—S) consisting of ten items is also available (Ventry & Weinstein, 1983; Weinstein, 1986).

Self-Assessment of Communication

The SAC (Schow & Nerbonne, 1982), which consists of ten items, was standardized on the basis of results for subjects whose ages ranged from 19 to 80 years. These items assess communication difficulties in various situations, clients' feelings about the handicap, and clients' perception of how their hearing is perceived by others. The Significant Other Assessment of Communication (SOAC) is a companion scale to the SAC, identical to it except that the behaviors and situations are rated by a SOP.

The Communication Profile for the Hearing Impaired

The CPHI (Demorest & Erdman, 1986; 1987) is designed to provide a comprehensive view of the difficulties encountered by people with hearing impairments. The CPHI was developed through research conducted with active and retired military personnel who had bilateral high-frequency sensorineural hearing losses and histories of noise exposure and other causes. The CPHI comprises 145 questions in five main areas: communication performance, communication importance, communication environment, communication strategies, and personal adjustment. There are 25 subscales within the five categories. Although the CPHI may prove a useful research tool for delineation of the problems of people with hearing impairments, its length and lack of normative data except for Walter Reed Army Hospital patients, make it fairly impractical for routine administration in the typical audiology practice.

The McCarthy-Alpiner Scale of Hearing Handicap

The McCarthy-Alpiner Scale of Hearing Handicap (M-A scale) (McCarthy & Alpiner, 1983) was developed to measure the psychologic, social, and vocational effects of hearing loss as reported by the person with the hearing impairment (form A) and by a family member (form B). Each form of the M-A scale consists of 34 reaction statements, which are rated on a scale from "always" to "never." A profile form is made into a graph after the scale is completed. The graph helps the audiologist determine if the hearing loss has affected the job, family, and social life of the person with the hearing impairment.

Performance Inventory for Profound and Severe Loss

The PIPSL (Owens & Raggio, 1988) is a 74-item self-rating inventory that samples perceived performance in a variety of communication situations and the reactions to these situations. It is particularly helpful for people with profound and severe hearing losses, for whom other assessment inventories may not be relevant.

Summary

Seven hearing handicap scales have been presented, by all means not a complete list. Selection of which scale to use depends on the audiologist's purpose for the assessment. The following guidelines are presented to simplify selection of the most appropriate scale.

Guidelines for Selection of a Hearing Scale

Purpose 1. Is there a significant hearing loss that indicates additional audiologic testing is necessary? Use the SAC or HHIE-S, because these scales were designed as short screening instruments to determine the need for further action.

Purpose 2: What are the patient's hearing care needs? Use any of the seven scales, because they were designed to identify the social and emotional effects that hearing impairment may have on a person.

Purpose 3. What is the efficacy of any treatment that may have been administered? It is difficult to provide guidelines in this area. The HHIE might be a good choice because it has undergone extensive standardization. However, Kricos et al (1992) expressed concern that some of the questions on the HHIE may not be sufficiently sensitive to indicate treatment efficacy. The training program used in their study focused on conversational strategies, empathic skills, and assertiveness training. Although conversational ease may have improved as a result of the 4-week communication training program, the improvement may not have been sufficient to reduce the perception of the overall handicap. For example, one of the HHIE questions asks whether a hearing problem causes feelings of frustration when talking to family members. It is doubtful that a 4-week communication training program will cause patients to no longer feel frustrated by their hearing losses, and therefore any benefits of the program may be masked. Kricos et al (1992) suggested that use of the HPI, with its detailed communication situation descriptors and five response options, might provide a more sensitive measurement than the HHIE. Both the HPI (Smaldino & Smaldino, 1988) and the HHIE (Abrams et al, 1992; Malinoff & Weinstein, 1989a,b; Mulrow et al, 1992; Newman & Weinstein, 1988) have been used, however, to document treatment efficacy.

Purpose 4. What are the family counseling needs of the person with the hearing impairment? Any of the scales described would be useful in identifying family counseling needs. Lending themselves most easily to couples counseling are the scales that have versions for both the person with the hearing impairment and the spouse or SOP. These include the HHIE, SAC-SOAC, and the M-A scale, all of which allow for direct comparison of responses from the hearing impaired person and the SOP.

EVALUATION OF COMMUNICATION SKILLS

An important part of the comprehensive care of an older adult is assessment of communication skills. By obtaining a profile of the communication abilities of a person with a hearing impairment, the audiologist can establish priorities about the communication needs of each patient. Four primary assessment areas to be described in this section are auditory speech reception, speechreading, audiovisual speech reception, and conversational fluency.

Auditory Speech Reception

Crandell (1991) and Helfer (1991) showed that a typical audiologic assessment does not give a complete or accurate representation of how older adults perform in everyday communication, especially when the audiologist is attempting to determine what rehabilitative strategies are needed. When possible, realistic listening conditions should be used, incorporating variables such as room acoustics (reverberation and noise), speech rate, message differences, and speaker differences. Henoch (1991) showed that most audiologists use lists of monosyllabic words to measure the speech discrimination abilities of their patients, despite the availability of a number of other measurements of speech intelligibility. Table 2–4 contains a summary of tests available to measure auditory speech reception. The protocol we recommend to obtain the most information in the least time is that proposed by Erber (1988).

Erber (1988) proposed evaluation of auditory speech reception in four areas: consonant identification; word identification; sentence identification; and identification of interactive sentences. For consonant identification, Erber (1988) recommended that auditory perception of consonants be screened with a small set of consonants, particularly ones that are frequently confused by people with significant hearing impairments. The Consonant Screening Test—Voice/Voiceless and Consonant Screening Test—Stop/Nasals based on Erber's suggestions can be found in Appendixes 2–4 and 2–5. These tests take only minutes to administer, and can provide useful information regarding the client's need for analytic training, speechreading instruction, and other rehabilitative strategies (Erber, 1988).

TABLE 2–4   Tests of Auditory Speech Reception

Test	Author/ References	Stimulus	Task	Noise Background	Features
Nonsense Syllable Test	Edgerton & Danhauer (1979)	Nonsense syllables	Open set recognition	Not considered essential	Can be administered rapidly
Speech Perception in Noise Test	Kalikow et al (1977);/ Bilger (1984); Rubinstein & Boothroyd (1987); Schum & Matthews (1992)	Sentences with high and low predictability	Repetition of final word in sentence	Multitalker, + 10 to 0 signal-to-noise ratio (S/N)	Assesses linguistic and acoustic effects
Central Institute for the Deaf Everyday Sentence Lists Test	Harris et al (1961);/ Kricos et al (1992)	Everyday sentences	Sentence repetition	Optional	Can be used in a variety of ways
Adaptive speech recognition procedures	Dirks et al (1982); Plomp & Mimpen (1979); Plomp (1986)	Usually sentences	Sentence repetition	S/N is varied to achieve 50 to 75 percent performance level	Can be used to assess effects of noise and reverberation
Synthetic Sentence Identification	Jerger & Hayes (1977)	Synthetic sentences	Sentence identification	S/N varies	Can be used to assess hearing aid benefit and to determine presence of central auditory disorder

TABLE 2–4   Tests of Auditory Speech Reception (continued)

Test	Author/ References	Stimulus	Task	Noise Background	Features
Connected Speech Test	Cox et al (1988)	10-sentence passages	Sentence repetition	Six-talker babble; varying S/N	Realistic message length; extensive standardiza- tion; avail- able in audiovisual format on laser video disk
California Consonant Test	Owens & Schubert (1977)	Words differing mainly in high-fre- quency discrimina- tion cues	Closed-set multiple- choice word dis- crimination	None	Helpful for consonant confusion identifica- tion
Minimal Auditory Capabilities Test	Owens et al (1981);/Fifer et al (1984)	Words and sentences	Varies with subtest; discrimina- tion; stimu- lus repetition	None	Subtests designed specifically for adults with severe hearing loss
Speech tracking	De Filippo & Scott (1978);/ Owens & Telleen (1981)	Groups of words (often prose)	Timed verbatim repetition	Optional	Provides quantifiable measure of communi- cation difficulties

To assess word identification, Erber (1988) suggested that conventional phonetically balanced word lists, scored in terms of proportion of phonemes correctly identified with auditory, visual, or auditory visual modes, be supplemented with high-frequency word lists. Erber's list of words containing high-frequency consonants can be found in Appendix 2–6.

Erber (1988) presents a unique protocol for sentence identification testing. Sentences such as the Central Institure for the Deaf Everyday Sentences (Harris et al, 1961) may be used, but each sentence is presented with modifications until the patient responds correctly. Erber (1988) suggested beginning with sentences that are spoken without acoustic cues then progressively adding cues as necessary. We suggest the opposite. The test should begin with presentations of a sentence with auditory cues only. If the person being tested responds correctly, the test proceeds to the next sentence. If the response is incorrect, subsequent presentations are given in the following order: repetition of sentence; repetition of sentence with increased clarity; repetition of sentence with visual cues for selected key words or phrases; repetition of the entire sentence with both auditory and visual cues. By noting the number of sentences identified correctly when each strategy is used, the audiologist will have useful information about what kinds of conditions are necessary for optimal speech reception by the patient. A recording form for the sentence identification test can be found in Appendix 2–7.

The rationale behind Erber's interactive sentence identification test is that in most conventional sentence identification procedures, patients assume a relatively passive role as they attempt to understand a series of unrelated sentences. Use of an interactive framework provides a more realistic representation of how the patient performs in real conversations. Erber's QUEST?AR uses a scripted set of questions about a recently made trip (eg, to the zoo, to Washington, DC). The patient asks the questions of the audiologist. For example, the patient may ask questions such as "Where did you go?" "How did you get there?" "What did you see along the way?" The QUEST?AR is available for purchase by writing: Norman P. Erber, Department of Communication Disorders, Lincoln Institute of Health Sciences, 625 Swanston Street, Carlton, Victoria 3053 Australia.

Speechreading

An excellent discussion of issues related to the evaluation of speechreading is contained in Montgomery and Demorest (1988). These authors emphasize the difficulties in developing an adequate measure of speechreading and encourage continued refinement of several innovative approaches to speechreading assessment. Table 2–5 contains a summary of some of the speechreading tests available. We recommend Erber's (1988) protocol for assessment of the visual perception of consonants (see Appendix 2–8 for the Lipreading Screening Test). This speechreading screening test can be administered quickly and is useful for identifying whether analytic practice might be beneficial or whether additional assessment (Table 2–5) is warranted.

Audiovisual Speech Reception

The ability to understand speech through a combination of aided hearing and speechreading is an important area of evaluation, although it is even more subject to procedural difficulties than the assessment of speechreading (Montgomery & Demorest, 1988). Table 2–6 contains a summary of ways to evaluate audiovisual speech reception.

TABLE 2–5 Speechreading Tests

Test	Author/References	Stimulus	Task	Features
Lipreading Discrimination Test	Bement et al (1988)	Sentences	Standard sentence versus comparison sentence discrimination	Allows assessment of viseme perception using sentences
Consonant Confusion Lip-reading Screening Test	Binnie et al (1976)	Consonants in syllables	Recognition of consonants within viseme groups	Provides rapid evaluation of viseme perception
Continuous Discourse Intelligibility Estimation Procedure	Hawkins et al (1988);/ Montgomery & Demorest (1988)	Continuous discourse	Estimate percentage of intelligibility as S/N varies	Allows comparison of Performance-Intensity functions of intelligibility estimations obtained with auditory only and auditory visual means; difference in S/N (auditory visual–auditory) is inferred visual benefit
Tracking	De Filippo & Scott (1978);/ Tye-Murray & Tyler (1988)	Groups of words (often prose)	Timed verbatim repetition	Provides quantifiable measurement of communication difficulties
Speechreading Test on the Utilization of Contextual Cues	Gagné et al (1991)	Introductory (captioned and spoken without sound) and test (spoken without sound) sentences	Write each test sentence (key words scored)	Assesses speechreader's ability to extract linguistic cues from a spoken message
Screening Visual Identification of Consonants	Erber (1988)	Eight consonants in /a/-C-/a/ context, presented five times	Consonant identification	Can be performed rapidly; delineates unusual speechreading errors that may be informative to the clinician

TABLE 2–6   Tests of Audiovisual Speech Reception

Test	Author	Stimulus	Task	Features
Garstecki Auditory-Visual Testing Paradigm	Garstecki (1981)	Utley sentences	Identification of sentences	Sentences presented in auditory visual condition, 72 dB sound pressure level (SPL) with 12 dB S/N; provides baseline for auditory-visual training paradigm
Nonsense Syllable Test	Edgerton & Danhauer (1979); Danhauer et al (1985)	Consonant-Vowel-Consonant-Vowel syllables	Syllable identification	Can be administered rapidly
Tracking	De Filippo & Scott (1978)	Typically continuous discourse	Timed verbatim repetition	Quantifiable measurement of communication difficulties
Connected Speech Test	Cox et al (1987; 1989)	10-sentence passages	Sentence repetition with key words scored	Realistic message length; extensive standardization; available on laser video disk

Conversational Fluency

Of all the communication skills to be assessed, undoubtedly the most important is the patient's conversational fluency. It is surprising that this area has received by far the least attention from researchers and practitioners. Table 2–7 contains a summary of possible evaluation tools for measuring conversational fluency. We have found Erber's (1988) TOPICON procedure to be useful in the subjective evaluation of a patient's overall conversational abilities. In brief, the patient and audiologist choose a topic of conversation and converse for 5 to 10 minutes, during which time auditory and visual distractions may be included as necessary. The conversational sample is evaluated by the clinician. The TOPICON rating scale in Appendix 2–9 is used to guide the clinician's subjective evaluation of the patient's conversational abilities. The scale allows assessment of degree of conversational fluency, the

TABLE 2–7 Measurements of Conversational Fluency

Test	Author	Task	Features
Continuous Discourse Tracking	De Filippo & Scott (1978)	Timed verbatim repetition of message, usually prose	Although not a direct conversational measure, allows inference of degree of conversational difficulty from the word-per-minute score and analysis of strategies used to resolve communication breakdown
Strategies Usage Test	Tye-Murray (1991)	Repetition of 20 sentences stored on video disk; selection of one of five repair strategies when verbatim repetition not possible	Provides record of which repair strategies (repeat, rephrase, simplify, key word, two sentences) patient is using
TOPICON	Erber (1988)	Engage in 5- to 10-minute conversation with clinician or SOP	Allows for subjective evaluation of conversational ease, effect of background distractions, use of repair strategies

patient's response to communication breakdowns, the patient's use of repair strategies, and factors that contributed to or impeded conversational fluency.

CONCLUSION

The purpose of assessment for audiologic rehabilitation should be to evaluate the functional ability of a person so that a treatment plan can be formulated. Several domains should be considered, including the physical, psychologic, social, and communication status of the person. When possible, clinical and environmental assessments should be performed, which may involve both formal and informal procedures. Considering the variety of factors that may affect function, no one standard approach can be recommended for all patients. Choice of procedures should be based on effectiveness and efficiency. In all cases, it is important to look beyond a person's hearing status.

REFERENCES

Abrams, H. B., Hnath-Chisolm, T., Guerreiro, S.M., & Ritterman, S.I. (1992). The effects of intervention strategy on self-perception of hearing handicap. *Ear and Hearing, 13,* 371-377.

American Academy of Audiology (1991). Task force on hearing impairment in aged people. *Audiology Today, 3,* 7.

ASHA Report (1992). Considerations in screening adults/older persons for handicapping hearing impairments. *ASHA, 34,* 81-87

Bement, L., Wallber, J., De Filippo, C., Bochner, J., & Garrison, W. (1988). A new protocol for assessing viseme perception in sentence context: The Lipreading Discrimination Test. *Ear and Hearing, 9,* 33-40.

Bilger, R.C. (1984). *Manual for the clinical use of the Speech Perception in Noise (SPIN) Test.* Champaign-Urbana: University of Illinois Press.

Binnie, C.A., Jackson, P.L., & Montgomery, A.A. (1976). Visual intelligibility of consonants: A lipreading screening test with implications for aural rehabilitation. *Journal of Speech and Hearing Disorders, 41,* 530-539.

Blazer, D., & Williams, C.D. (1980). Epidemiology of dysphoria and depression in an elderly population. *American Journal of Psychiatry, 37,* 439-444.

Cadieux, R.J., Kales, J.D., & Zimmerman, L. (1985). Comprehensive assessment of the elderly patient. *American Family Physician, 31,* 105-111.

Cox, R.M., Alexander, G.C., & Gilmore, C. (1987). Development of the Connected Speech Test (CST). *Ear and Hearing, 8* (Suppl.), 119S-126S.

Cox, R.M., Alexander, G.C., Gilmore, C. & Pusakulich, K.M. (1988). Use of the Connected Speech Test (CST) with hearing-impaired listeners. *Ear and Hearing, 9,* 198-207.

Cox, R.C., Alexander, G.C., Gilmore, C., & Pusakulich, K.M. (1989). The Connected Speech Test Version 3: Audiovisual administration. *Ear and Hearing, 10,* 29-32.

Crandell, C.C. (1991). Individual differences in speech recognition ability: Implications for hearing aid selection. *Ear and Hearing, 12,* 100S-108S.

Danhauer, J.L., Garnett, C.M., & Edgerton, B.J. (1985). Older person's performance on auditory, visual, and auditory-visual presentations of the Edgerton and Danhauer Nonsense Syllable Test. *Ear and Hearing, 6,* 191-197.

De Filippo, C.L., & Scott, B.L. (1978). A method for training and evaluating the reception of ongoing speech. *Journal of the Acoustical Society of America, 63,* 1186-1192.

Demorest, M.E., & Erdman, S.A. (1986). Scale composition and item analysis of the Communication Profile for the Hearing Impaired. *Journal of Speech and Hearing Research, 29,* 515-535.

Demorest, M.E., & Erdman, S.A. (1987). Development of the Communication Profile for the Hearing Impaired. *Journal of Speech and Hearing Disorders, 52,* 129-139.

Dirks, D., Morgan, D., & Dubno, J. (1982). A procedure for quantifying the effects of noise on speech recognition. *Journal of Speech and Hearing Disorders, 47,* 114–123.

Edgerton, B.J., & Danhauer, J.L (1979). *Clinical implications of a speech discrimination test using nonsense stimuli.* Baltimore: University Park Press.

Erber, N.P. (1988). *Communication therapy for hearing-impaired adults.* Washington: Alexander Graham Bell Association for the Deaf.

Fifer, R.C., Stach, B.A., & Jerger, J.J. (1984). Evaluation of the Minimal Auditory Capabilities (MAC) Test in prelingual and postlingual hearing-impaired adults. *Ear and Hearing, 5,* 87-90.

Folstein, M.F., Folstein, S.E., & McHugh, P.R. (1975). "Mini-Mental State": A practical method for grading the cognitive state of patients for the clinician. *Journal of Psychiatric Research, 12,* 189-198.

Gagné, J.P., Tugby, K.G., & Michaud, J. (1991). Development of a speechreading test on the utilization of contextual cues (STUCC): Preliminary findings with normal-hearing subjects. *Journal of the Academy of Rehabilitative Audiology, 24,* 157-170.

Gallo, J.J., Reichel, W., & Andersen, L. (1988). *Handbook of geriatric assessment.* Rockville: Aspen.

Garstecki, D.C. (1981). Auditory, visual, and combined auditory-visual speech perception. *Journal of the Academy of Rehabilitative Audiology, 14,* 223-238.

Giolas, T.G., Owens, E., Lamb, S.H., & Schubert, E.D. (1979). Hearing performance inventory. *Journal of Speech and Hearing Disorders, 44,* 169-195.

Goldstein, D.P., & Stephens, S.D.G. (1981). Audiological rehabilitation: Management model I. *Audiology, 20,* 432-452.

Hardick, E.J., Oyer, H.J., & Irion, P.E. (1970). Lipreading performance as related to measurements of vision. *Journal of Speech and Hearing Research, 13,* 92-100.

Harris, J., Haines, H., Kelsey, P., & Clack, T. (1961). The relation between speech intelligibility and electroacoustic characteristics of low fidelity circuitry. *Journal of Audiological Research, 1,* 357-381.

Hartke, R.J. (1991) Introduction. In R.J. Hartke (Ed.), *Psychological aspects of geriatric rehabilitation* (pp. 1-8). Gaithersburg: Aspen.

Hawkins, D.B., Montgomery, A.A., Mueller, H.G., & Sedge, R.K. (1988). Assessment of speech intelligibility by hearing-impaired listeners. In B. Berglund, U. Berglund, J. Karlson & T. Lindvall (Eds.), *Noise as a public noise source* (vol. 2) (pp. 241-246). Stockholm: Swedish Council for Building Research.

Helfer, K.S. (1991). Everyday speech understanding by older listeners. *Journal of the Academy of Rehabilitative Audiology, 24,* 17-34.

Henoch, M. (1991). Speech perception, hearing aid technology, and aural rehabilitation: A future perspective. *Ear and Hearing, 12,* 1875-1915.

Herkind, P, Priest, R.S., & Schiller, G. (1983). *Compendium of ophthalmology.* Philadelphia: Lippincott.

Hiatt, L.G. (1990). Environmental factors in rehabilitation of disabled elderly people. In S.J. Brody & L.G. Pawlson (Eds.), *Aging and rehabilitation II: The state of the practice* (pp. 150-164). New York: Springer Publishing.

Jerger, J., & Hayes, D. (1977). Diagnostic speech audiometry. *Archives of Otolaryngology, 102,* 216-222.

Kalikow, D.N., Stevens, K.N., & Elliott, L.L. (1977). Development of a test of speech intelligibility in noise using sentence materials with controlled word predictability. *Journal of the Acoustical Society of America, 61,* 1337-1351.

Kane, R.L. (1990). Targeting geriatric assessment. In S.J. Brody & L.G. Pawlson (Eds.), *Aging and rehabilitation II: The state of the practice* (pp. 301-311). New York: Springer Publishing.

Kemp, B. (1986). Psychosocial and mental health issues in rehabilitation of older persons. In S.J. Brody & G.E. Ruff (Eds.), *Aging and rehabilitation: Advances in the state of the art* (pp. 122-158). New York: Springer Publishing.

Kemp, B. (1990). Motivational dynamics in geriatric rehabilitation toward a therapeutic model. In B. Kemp, K. Smith, & J. Ramsdell (Eds.), *Geriatric rehabilitation.* Boston: College Hill Press.

Kricos, P.B., Holmes, A.E., & Doyle, D.A. (1992). Efficacy of an auditory training program for hearing impaired elderly adults. *Journal of the Academy of Rehabilitative Audiology, 25,* 69-81.

Lachs, M.S., Feinstein, A.R., Cooney, L.M., et al (1990). A simple procedure for general screening for functional disability in elderly patients. *Annals of Internal Medicine, 112,* 699-706.

LaFerle, K.R., & LaFerle, I.A. (1988). Senility and its impact on the hearing instrument delivery session. *Hearing Instruments, 39,* 32-34.

Lichtenstein, M.J., Bess, F.H., & Logan, S.A. (1988). Validation of screening tools for identifying hearing impaired elderly in primary care. *JAMA, 259,* 2875-2878.

Lubinski, R. (1984). The environmental role in communication skills and opportunities of older people. In C. Wilder & B. Weinstein (Eds.), *Aging and communication: Problems in management* (pp. 47-57). New York: Haworth Press.

Malinoff, R.L., & Weinstein, B.E. (1989a). Measurement of hearing aid benefit in the elderly. *Ear and Hearing, 10,* 354-357.

Malinoff, R.L., & Weinstein, B.E. (1989b). Changes in self-assessment of hearing handicap over the first year of hearing aid use by older adults. *Journal of the Academy of Rehabilitative Audiology, 22,* 54-61.

McCarthy, P., & Alpiner, J. (1983). An assessment scale of hearing handicap for use in family counseling. *Journal of the Academy of Rehabilitative Audiology, 16,* 256-271.

McCarthy, P.A., Montgomery, A.A., & Mueller, H.G. (1990). Decision making in rehabilitative audiology. *Journal of the American Academy of Audiology, 1,* 23-30.

Montgomery, A.A., & Demorest, M.E. (1988). Issues and development in the evaluation of speechreading. *Volta Review, 90,* 193-215.

Morgan, A.C. (1989). Special issues of assessment and treatment of suicide risk in the elderly. In D. Jacobs & H.N. Brown (Eds.), *Suicide: Understanding and responding* (pp. 239-255). Madison: International Universities Press.

Mulrow, C.D., Tuley, M.R., & Aguilar, C. (1992). Sustained benefits of hearing aids. *Journal of Speech and Hearing Research, 35,* 1402-1405.

National Center for Health Statistics (1987). Current estimates from the National Health Interview Survey: United States, 1987. Vital and Health Statistics. Series 10. Public Health Service, Washington: United States Government Printing Office.

Newman, C., & Weinstein, B. (1988). The hearing handicap inventory for the elderly as a measure of hearing aid benefit. *Ear and Hearing, 9,* 81-85.

Owens, E.D., Kessler, D., Telleen, C., & Schubert, E. (1981). The minimal auditory capabilities (MAC) battery. *Hearing Journal, 34,* 32-34.

Owens, E., & Raggio, M. (1988). Performance inventory for profound and severe loss (PIPSL). *Journal of Speech and Hearing Disorders, 53*, 42-56.

Owens, E., & Schubert, E.D. (1977). Development of the California Consonant Test. *Journal of Speech and Hearing Research, 20*, 463-474.

Owens, E., & Telleen, C.C. (1981). Tracking as an aural rehabilitative process. *Journal of the Academy of Rehabilitative Audiology, 14*, 252-258.

Palmer, C. (1992). Computer administration of hearing performance inventories. *American Journal of Audiology, 1*, 13-14.

Pfeiffer, E. (1975). A short portable mental status questionnaire for the assessment of organic brain deficit in elderly patients. *Journal of the American Geriatric Society, 23*, 433-441.

Piercy, S.K., & Goldstein, D.P. (1994). Hearing aid rejection: The type III individual. *ASHA, 36*, 51-52.

Plomp, R. (1986). A signal-to-noise ratio model for the speech reception threshold of the hearing impaired. *Journal of Speech and Hearing Research, 29*, 146-154.

Plomp, R., & Mimpen, A. (1979). Improving the reliability of testing the speech reception threshold for sentences. *Audiology, 18*, 43-52.

Richman, J. (1991). Suicide and the elderly. In A.A. Leenaars (Ed.), *Life span perspectives of suicide* (pp. 153-167). New York: Plenum.

Ross, M. (1987). Aural rehabilitation revisited. *Journal of the Academy of Rehabilitative Audiology, 20*, 13-23.

Roth, E.J. (1991). The aging process: Physiological changes. In R.J. Hartke (Ed.), *Psychological aspects of geriatric rehabilitation* (pp. 9-41). Gaithersburg: Aspen.

Rubinstein, A., & Boothroyd, A. (1987). Effect of two approaches to auditory training on speech recognition by hearing-impaired adults. *Journal of Speech and Hearing Research, 30*, 153-160.

Schow, R., & Nerbonne, M. (1982). Communication screening profile uses with elderly clients. *Ear and Hearing, 3*, 133-147.

Schum, D.J., & Matthews, L.J. (1992). SPIN Test performance of elderly hearing-impaired listeners. *Journal of the American Academy of Audiology, 3*, 303-307.

Shadden, B.B. (1988). Education, counseling, and support for significant others. In B.B. Shadden (Ed.), *Communication behavior and aging: A sourcebook for clinicians* (pp. 309-328). Baltimore: Williams & Wilkins.

Smaldino, S.E., & Smaldino, J.J. (1988). The influence of aural rehabilitation and cognitive style disclosure on the perception of hearing handicap. *Journal of the Academy of Rehabilitative Audiology, 21*, 54-67.

Trezona, R.R. (1991). The assessment of rehabilitation potential: Emotional factors. In R.J. Hartke (Ed.), *Psychological aspects of geriatric rehabilitation* (pp. 115-134). Gaithersburg: Aspen.

Tye-Murray, N. (1991). Repair strategy usage by hearing-impaired adults and changes following communication therapy. *Journal of Speech and Hearing Research, 34*, 921-928.

Tye-Murray, N., & Tyler, R.S. (1988). A critique of continuous discourse tracking as a test procedure. *Journal of Speech and Hearing Disorders, 53*, 226-251.

Ventry, I.M., & Weinstein, B.E. (1982). The hearing handicap inventory for the elderly: A new tool. *Ear and Hearing, 3*, 128-133.

Ventry, I., & Weinstein, B. (1983). Identification of elderly people with hearing problems. *ASHA, 25*, 37-47.

Weinstein, B. (1986). Validity of a screening protocol for identifying elderly people with hearing problems. *ASHA, 28*, 41-45.

Yesavage, J.A., & Brink, T.L. (1983). Development and validation of a geriatric depression screening scale: A preliminary report. *Journal of Psychiatric Research, 17*, 37-49.

Appendix 2–1

Global Assessment Domains, Procedures, and Rehabilitative Implications

Domain	Informal Assessment	Formal Assessment	Rehabilitative Implications
General health	Ask: "Are you experiencing any health problems? Ask: "Are you taking any medication?"		(1) Modify treatment, treatment milieu, or scheduling, as necessary. (2) Make necessary referrals.
Vision	Ask: "Are you having any difficulty seeing?"	Test aided binocular acuity with Snellen chart, Jaeger card, or other vision screening technique.	(1) Encourage the use of spectacles, if indicated. (2) Make necessary changes in or substitutions for written therapy materials. (3) Provide preferential seating or assistance during treatment. (4) Modify environment to maximize visual reception. (5) Provide referral to vision care specialist.

Domain	Informal Assessment	Formal Assessment	Rehabilitative Implications
Dexterity and fine motor skills	Proximal: Observe as patient lifts hearing aid to ear. Distal: Observe as patient manipulates hearing aid battery.		(1) Make appropriate modifications in prosthetic devices. (2) Enlist the assistance of a SOP. (3) Provide repeated learning opportunities. (4) Provide referral to physical or occupational therapist.
Mental status	Observe affect, orientation, memory, and judgment, especially calculational abilities and short-term memory.	Administer "Short Portable Mental Status Questionnaire" or Folstein "Mini-Mental Status Examination."	(1) Enlist the assistance of a SOP. (2) Provide repeated learning opportunities. (3) Provide medical referral.
Motivation	On the basis of interview and observation, determine the patient's wants, beliefs, potential rewards, and the physical, economic, emotional, and social costs.		(1) Provide counseling. 2) Encourage the development of realistic expectations.
Attitude	On the basis of observation and interview, classify patient as Type I, II, III, or IV.		(1) Encourage participation in an auditory rehabilitation program (a group program is especially useful for Type III patients). (2) Provide support, patience, and encouragement.

Domain	Informal Assessment	Formal Assessment	Rehabilitative Implications
Depression	Ask: "Do you often feel sad or depressed?"	Administer "Geriatric Depression Scale."	(1) Provide referral to mental health or medical personnel. (2) Encourage participation in an individualized therapy program.
Social environment	Identify, on the basis of ecologic assessment if possible, SOPs or people with whom the patient interacts and experiences communication difficulties.		(1) Encourage participation of a SOP in a group auditory rehabilitation program or individualized therapy. (2) Provide suggestions for behavioral modifications. (3) Explore the use of assistive listening devices.
Physical environment	Identify, on the basis of ecologic assessment, difficult situations and possible intervention strategies.		(1) Explore the use of assistive listening devices. (2) Recommend needed environmental modifications. (3) Provide suggestions for behavioral modifications.

Appendix 2–2

The Hearing Handicap Inventory for the Elderly

Instructions: The purpose of this scale is to identify the problems your hearing loss may be causing you. Check YES, SOMETIMES, or NO for each question. Do not skip a question if you avoid a situation because of your hearing problem. If you use a hearing aid, please answer the way you hear without the aid.

		YES (4)	SOME-TIMES (2)	NO (0)
S-1	Does a hearing problem cause you to use the phone less often than you would like?	___	___	___
E-2	Does a hearing problem cause you to feel embarrassed when meeting new people?	___	___	___
S-3	Does a hearing problem cause you to avoid groups of people?	___	___	___
E-4	Does a hearing problem make you irritable?	___	___	___
E-5	Does a hearing problem cause you to feel frustrated when talking to members of your family?	___	___	___
S-6	Does a hearing problem cause you difficulty when attending a party?	___	___	___
E-7	Does a hearing problem cause you to feel "stupid" or "dumb"?	___	___	___
S-8	Do you have difficulty hearing when someone speaks in a whisper?	___	___	___
E-9	Do you feel handicapped by a hearing problem?	___	___	___
S-10	Does a hearing problem cause you difficulty when visiting friends, relatives, or neighbors?	___	___	___
S-11	Does a hearing problem cause you to attend religious services less often than you would like?	___	___	___

	YES (4)	SOME-TIMES (2)	NO (0)
E-12 Does a hearing problem cause you to be nervous?	——	——	——
S-13 Does a hearing problem cause you to visit friends, relatives, or neighbors less often than you would like?	——	——	——
E-14 Does a hearing problem cause you to have arguments with family members?	——	——	——
S-15 Does a hearing problem cause you difficulty when listening to television or radio?	——	——	——
S-16 Does a hearing problem cause you to go shopping less often than you would like?	——	——	——
E-17 Does any problem or difficulty with your hearing upset you at all?	——	——	——
E-18 Does a hearing problem cause you to want to be by yourself?	——	——	——
S-19 Does a hearing problem cause you to talk to family members less often than you would like?	——	——	——
E-20 Do you feel that any difficulty with your hearing limits or hampers your personal or social life?	——	——	——
S-21 Does a hearing problem cause you difficulty when in a restaurant with relatives or friends?	——	——	——
E-22 Does a hearing problem cause you to feel depressed?	——	——	——
S-23 Does a hearing problem cause you to listen to television or radio less often than you would like?	——	——	——
E-24 Does a hearing problem cause you to feel uncomfortable when talking to friends?	——	——	——
E-25 Does a hearing problem cause you to feel left out when you are with a group of people?	——	——	——

FOR CLINICIAN'S USE ONLY:

Total Score: ——
Subtotal E: ——
Subtotal S: ——

(Reprinted with permission from Ventry & Weinstein 1982).

Appendix 2–3

Self-Assessment of Communication

Name _____ Date_____

Raw Score _____ × 2 = _____ − 20 = _____ × 1.25 _____%

Please select the appropriate number ranging from 1 to 5 for the following questions. Circle only one number for each question. If you have a hearing aid, please fill out the form according to how you communicate when the hearing aid is in use.

Various Communication Situations

1. Do you experience communication difficulties in situations when speaking with one other person? (eg, at home, at work, in a social situation, with a waitress, a store clerk, with a spouse, boss, etc.)

    (1) almost never or never
    (2) occasionally (about one-fourth of the time)
    (3) about half of the time
    (4) frequently (about three-fourths of the time)
    (5) practically always or always

2. Do you experience communication difficulties in situations when conversing with a small group of several persons? (eg, with friends or family, co-workers, in meetings or casual conversations, over dinner or while playing cards)

    (1) almost never or never
    (2) occasionally (about one-fourth of the time)
    (3) about half of the time
    (4) frequently (about three-fourths of the time)
    (5) practically always or always

3. Do you experience communication difficulties while listening to some-one speak to a large group? (eg, at church or in a civic meeting, at a club, at an educational lecture)

   (1) almost never or never
   (2) occasionally (about one-fourth of the time)
   (3) about half of the time
   (4) frequently (about three-fourths of the time)
   (5) practically always or always

4. Do you experience communication difficulties while participating in various types of entertainment? (eg, movies, television, radio, plays, night clubs, musical entertainment)

   (1) almost never or never
   (2) occasionally (about one-fourth of the time)
   (3) about half of the time
   (4) frequently (about three-fourths of the time)
   (5) practically always or always

5. Do you experience communication difficulties when you are in an un-favorable listening environment? (eg, at a noisy party, where there is background music, when riding in a car or bus, when someone whis-pers or talks from across the room)

   (1) almost never or never
   (2) occasionally (about one-fourth of the time)
   (3) about half of the time
   (4) frequently (about three-fourths of the time)
   (5) practically always or always

6. Do you experience communication difficulties when using or listening to various communication devices? (eg, telephone, telephone ring, doorbell, public address system, warning signals, alarms)

   (1) almost never or never
   (2) occasionally (about one-fourth of the time)
   (3) about half of the time
   (4) frequently (about three-fourths of the time)
   (5) practically always or always

Feelings About Communication

7. Do you feel that any difficulty with your hearing limits or hampers your personal or social life?

    (1) almost never or never

    (2) occasionally (about one-fourth of the time)

    (3) about half of the time

    (4) frequently (about three-fourths of the time)

    (5) practically always or always

8. Does any problem or difficulty with your hearing upset you?

    (1) almost never or never

    (2) occasionally (about one-fourth of the time)

    (3) about half of the time

    (4) frequently (about three-fourths of the time)

    (5) practically always or always

Other People

9. Do others suggest that you have a hearing problem?

    (1) almost never or never

    (2) occasionally (about one-fourth of the time)

    (3) about half of the time

    (4) frequently (about three-fourths of the time)

    (5) practically always or always

10. Do others leave you out of conversations or become annoyed because of your hearing?

    (1) almost never or never

    (2) occasionally (about one-fourth of the time)

    (3) about half of the time

    (4) frequently (about three-fourths of the time)

    (5) practically always or always

(Reprinted with permission from Schow & Nerbonne 1982)

Appendix 2–4

Consonant Screening Test — Voice/Voiceless

Present the following consonants in an /a/-C-/a/ context:

1. v ___	9. /3/ ___	17. th ___	25. sh ___
2. sh ___	10. s ___	18. TH ___	26. f ___
3. f ___	11. TH ___	19. z ___	27. /3/ ___
4. s ___	12. v ___	20. f ___	28. TH ___
5. th ___	13. z ___	21. /3/ ___	29. s ___
6. z ___	14. f ___	22. v ___	30. th ___
7. /3/ ___	15. sh ___	23. sh ___	31. z ___
8. TH ___	16. th ___	24. s ___	32. v ___

		Stimulus							
		f	th	sh	s	v	TH	/3/	z
	f								
	th								
	sh								
Response	s								
	v								
	TH								
	/3/								
	z								

(Adapted from Erber 1988)

53

Appendix 2–5

Consonant Screening Test — Stop/Nasals

Present the following consonants in an /a/-C-/a/ context:

1. t ___	9. n ___	17. b ___	25. g ___
2. m ___	10. d ___	18. t ___	26. m ___
3. p ___	11. m ___	19. g ___	27. k ___
4. d ___	12. p ___	20. k ___	28. b ___
5. k ___	13. t ___	21. p ___	29. p ___
6. n ___	14. k ___	22. l ___	30. t ___
7. g ___	15. b ___	23. m ___	31. d ___
8. b ___	16. g ___	24. d ___	32. n ___

Stimulus

	p	t	k	b	d	g	m	n
p								
t								
k								
Response b								
d								
g								
m								
v								

(Adapted from Erber 1988)

Appendix 2–6

High Frequency Word Lists

kit	shipped	sips	sits	pick
sticks	fists	kissed	picked	thick
ticked	chicks	fist	sip	fixed
stiff	tips	skipped	fits	chips
fit	spit	kick	pitch	kiss
chip	fish	picks	chipped	sipped
fished	pit	spits	stick	ships
kicks	skip	tipped	kits	tip
sick	kicked	ship	fix	sit
pits	six	chick	tick	skips

(Reprinted with permission from Erber 1988)

Appendix 2–7

Sentence Identification

Use 20 everyday sentences (eg, those from Harris et al, 1961). Present each sentence until it is correctly identified. Each time a sentence is missed, modify it according to this hierarchy:

1. Original presentation (auditory only)
2. Repetition of sentence (auditory only)
3. Repetition with increased clarity (slight exaggeration; auditory only)
4. Repetition with visual (lipreading) cues for selected key words or phrases
5. Repetition of entire sentence with simultaneous auditory and visual cues.

Record Results Below:

	Number of Sentences Correct
Auditory only	_____
Repetition	_____
Exaggeration	_____
Auditory plus lipreading key word	_____
Auditory and visual cues for entire sentence	_____
	_____
Total	_____ /20

(Adapted from Erber 1988)

Appendix 2–8

Lipreading Screening Test

Name _____   Date_____

Amplification _____

Present the following consonants in an /a/-C-/a/ context:

1. v ___	11. /dʒ/ ___	21. l ___	31. g ___
2. d ___	12. b ___	22. d ___	32. v ___
3. l ___	13. TH ___	23. l ___	33. /dʒ/ ___
4. /dʒ/ ___	14. g ___	24. /dʒ/ ___	34. g ___
5. b ___	15. d ___	25. w ___	35. w ___
6. g ___	16. w ___	26. g ___	36. d ___
7. TH ___	17. v ___	27. v ___	37. b ___
8. w ___	18. /dʒ/ ___	28. l ___	38. l ___
9. b ___	19. TH ___	29. d ___	39. v ___
10. TH ___	20. w ___	30. b ___	40. TH ___

Stimulus

	/dʒ/	w	b	v	TH	l	d	g
/dʒ/								
w								
b								
Response v								
TH								
l								
d								
g								

(Adapted from Erber 1988)

57

Appendix 2–9

TOPICON Rating Sheet

Topic: _____

		Clinician	
		Low	High
Topic Familiarity:	*Client*	Low ___	___
		High ___	___

Rating

Low ___ ___ ___ ___ High

Overall fluency of discourse:
Factors related to fluency:

a. presupposition   ___ ___ ___ ___ ___
b. receptive abilities (auditory, visual,
   auditory visual)   ___ ___ ___ ___ ___
c. expressive abilities   ___ ___ ___ ___ ___
d. motivation, attention   ___ ___ ___ ___ ___
e. turn taking   ___ ___ ___ ___ ___
f. specificity, accuracy   ___ ___ ___ ___ ___
g. new versus old information   ___ ___ ___ ___ ___
h. nonverbal communication   ___ ___ ___ ___ ___
i. topic maintenance   ___ ___ ___ ___ ___
j. cooperation   ___ ___ ___ ___ ___
k. time sharing   ___ ___ ___ ___ ___
l. verification   ___ ___ ___ ___ ___
m. independent repair   ___ ___ ___ ___ ___
n. metacommunication   ___ ___ ___ ___ ___
o. other _____   ___ ___ ___ ___ ___
Comments:

_____
_____

(Reprinted with permission from Erber 1988)

Chapter 3

Hearing Aids and the Older Adult

Alice E. Holmes

Hearing aids are the primary rehabilitative tools audiologists have to offer older adults with hearing losses (Bess et al, 1990). The benefits of hearing aids in the older adult population are well documented (Harless & McConnell, 1982; Kricos et al, 1987; Malinoff & Weinstein, 1989; Mulrow et al, 1990; Newman et al, 1991; Taylor, 1993). Self-perceived hearing handicaps were shown to be considerably reduced after only 3 weeks of hearing-aid use by 92 percent of elderly adults with hearing losses who had not previously worn amplification (Newman et al, 1991). Taylor (1993) used the Hearing Handicap Inventory for the Elderly—Screening Version (HHIE-S) (Ventry & Weinstein, 1983) to study this reduction in self-perceived handicap over the first year of hearing-aid use by 58 elderly people. Substantial reduction in handicap was found 3 weeks, 3 months, 6 months, and 1 year after fitting. The improvement was most pronounced 3 months after fitting and stabilized to clinically significant although was not as dramatic an improvement for the other measurement intervals.

The American Association of Retired Persons (AARP) reported that although most people with hearing impairments receive a substantial benefit from the use of hearing aids, more than three-fourths of those who need amplification do not use hearing aids (Gabbard, 1994). In 1989, nearly 61 percent of the hearing aids sold were to elderly patients, yet estimates suggest that only about 18 to 25 percent of the older population with hearing losses own hearing aids (Davis & Mueller, 1987; Gallup, 1980). Schow (1982) reported that only about 10 percent of the nursing home population with hearing losses 40 decibels hearing level (dB HL) or greater used hearing aids. Thibodeau and Schmitt (1988) evaluated hearing aids in 17 nursing homes and three retirement centers. They found that only 4 percent of the 493 nursing home residents and 5 percent of the 451 retirement center residents used amplification. Older people do not obtain hearing aids for a number of reasons, including attitudes, motivation, prior direct and indirect experience, financial resources, and self-perceived handicap.

ATTITUDES TOWARD HEARING AIDS

Acceptance or rejection of amplification by the elderly population is affected greatly by their attitudes and expectations about the possible benefits and limitations of hearing aids. Kricos et al (1991) administered a questionnaire dealing with expectations regarding hearing aids to 100 older adults who had never worn amplification. In general, the subjects in the study were very positive toward hearing aids. Eighty-seven percent had medium to high expectations for hearing-aid use. These results should be both promising and worrisome to audiologists. Whereas positive expectations could influence people with hearing losses to seek amplification, these patients may ultimately reject their hearing aids if their expectations are not met. The importance of counseling patients on both the benefits and limitations of hearing aids cannot be overemphasized.

Franks and Beckman (1985) surveyed 100 older adults (50 hearing-aid users and 50 who did not wear hearing aids) on their attitudes toward hearing aids. More than 70 percent of the respondents believed hearing aids cost too much and that they call attention to the handicap. Worries over dealers' sales practices and training were expressed. Of the ten most frequent concerns respondents had about hearing aids, only two dealt with the actual quality of the sound from hearing aids. Fifty-seven percent of the respondents said that hearing aids amplify noise, and 49 percent were concerned about sounds being too loud. The other ten factors dealt with appearance, convenience, and selling issues.

In another study, 490 elderly users of hearing aids were given the opportunity to respond to an open-ended question about their hearing aids (Smedley & Schow, 1994). Of 406 comments received, 64 percent were negative, 14 percent positive, and 22 percent informational. The negative issues reported included difficulties in noise and groups (28 percent); fitting, comfort, and mechanical problems (25 percent); too little benefit (18 percent); and cost (17 percent).

Attitudes toward the visibility of hearing aids have been emphasized both in the research literature and in consumer advertisements. The results of one study suggested that people have negative biases toward older users of hearing aids (Johnson et al, 1982). Iler et al (1982), however, found that geriatric peers did not have negative biases toward older users of hearing aids. Smaller, less visible hearing aids are promoted to the public by many manufacturers as mitigating the problem of negative attitudes about hearing-aid use.

Attitudes of various health care professionals need to be considered when working with the older population. Unfortunately, many professionals are unaware of changes in hearing health care and in modern hearing-aid technology. Some patients still report that they were told they could not benefit from hearing aids because they had "nerve deafness." Audiologists must help inform other health care professionals about the availability of and necessity for audiologic services among the elderly population (Shadden & Raiford, 1984). In particular, primary care physicians must be educated about the effects of hearing loss on the quality of life of older patients. When a patient describes reduced hearing to a physician, there is only a 50 percent chance that the physician will provide a referral for audiologic rehabilitation (Bess et al, 1987).

The problems and frustrations that hearing impairment can cause are not always evident to the public. Unfortunately, most information consumers receive about hearing loss and hearing aids comes from television, radio, newspaper, or magazine advertisements and from acquaintances. This information often can be misleading. Public education is needed to provide accurate information on hearing loss and hearing aids.

HEARING-AID CANDIDACY

Many factors need to be considered in deciding if an older person is a candidate for hearing-aid use. A pure-tone audiogram alone is not a good predictor of success with amplification. In a study of 176 veterans, a number of both demographic and clinical variables were investigated to find predictive value for hearing-aid use (Mulrow et al, 1992). Several variables were found to have a statistically significant correlation with successful hearing-aid use. These variables included greater self-perceived handicap, younger age, lower educational levels, use of fewer medications, better vision, more high-frequency gain, and less speech recognition threshold gain. Although the variance associated with these variables could not be used to predict success, the variables should be considered in the counseling of prospective users of hearing aids.

Fino et al (1992) investigated acceptance of hearing aids in a group of older people referred for audiologic follow-up evaluations. These patients were referred after failing a hearing screening at 40 dB HL in their physician's office. Of the 178 patients who were referred, 83 were determined to be candidates for hearing-aid use on the basis of audiometric results. Of these patients 14 already had hearing aids and 11 chose to purchase them. The remaining 58 patients declined hearing aids. Most of the patients who rejected hearing aids indicated it was because of the cost or because they considered hearing aids too conspicuous.

A number of studies with elderly people have suggested a relation between age and successful use of a hearing aid (Brooks, 1985; 1989; Mulrow et al, 1992). These studies indicated a decline in use as a person gets older. Other investigators did not find this age relationship. Davis and Mueller (1987) found similar satisfaction, benefit, and use among patients older than and younger than 70 years.

Parving and Phillip (1991) surveyed 139 users of hearing aids 90 years of age and older. They found that 76 percent used their hearing aids at home,

33 percent used them in large group situations, and 17 percent used them in the theater. Fifty-three percent of these elders used their hearing aids on a daily basis. The authors found a high rate of handling problems, particularly among new users. Only 44 percent of first-time users of hearing aids could insert their aids themselves compared with 75 percent of previous users.

HEARING-AID SELECTION AND FITTING

Numerous books and articles are available on conventional selection and fitting procedures for adults with hearing losses. Techniques do not differ greatly for older adults, although some modifications of traditional approaches need to be considered. Some studies have indicated that elderly users of hearing aids require less gain than younger users (Humes & Kirn, 1990; Leijon et al, 1984). Choosing a prescriptive formula with less gain, such as that of the Revised National Acoustic Laboratories (R-NAL) (Byrne & Dillon, 1986) may be preferable for the older population. Ryals and Auther (1990), using several different formulas, found no difference between older and younger patients in their preferred hearing-aid gain, but aids that provided less insertion gain were preferred by both groups.

CENTRAL AUDITORY PROCESSING DISORDERS

Audiologists should be aware of the complex nature of hearing loss in the elderly when evaluating and fitting them with hearing aids. Hearing loss in the elderly often involves a central as well as a peripheral hearing loss. This central auditory processing disorder (CAPD) can cause decreased speech perception abilities, especially in difficult listening situations, such as noisy environments. Stach et al (1990) estimated that 58 percent of clinic patients 65 to 70 years of age with hearing losses have a CAPD. The rate increases to 95 percent for patients 80 years and older age. Some researchers have stated that people with CAPDs are less likely to receive benefits from conventional analog hearing aids (Hayes & Jerger, 1979; Stach, 1990).

Kricos et al (1987), on the other hand, measured the perceived benefit of hearing-aid use in 24 older adults with sensorineural hearing loss (10 peripheral and 14 CAPD). They found no relation between the perceived benefit of hearing-aid use and central auditory function. Therefore, if an older person has a central component to the hearing loss, amplification can be recommended, although careful counseling is required to ensure that the person has realistic expectations about the use of hearing aids.

Hearing-aid modifications and options that minimize the effects of background noise should be considered for elderly patients. Directional microphones and the use of binaural hearing aids can improve speech recognition in noise. Advances in the signal processing of hearing aids may prove to be effective in amplification for elderly people with hearing losses and CAPD (Crandell, 1991). A number of programmable hearing aids offer adaptive features for compression, noise suppression, and filtering. Caution should be taken not to overload the user with too many controls or settings on the aids. Gordon-Salant and Sherlock (1992) evaluated the use of adaptive frequency response (AFR) circuitry in 10 older adults with hearing losses. They found that the subjects performed better on the high-predictability items of the Revised Speech Perception in Noise test (R-SPIN) when they used AFR hearing aids.

ONE AID OR TWO?

People with bilateral symmetric hearing losses usually benefit more from the use of binaural amplification than from the use of one hearing aid. Increased localization abilities (Byrne et al, 1992) and improved speech recognition in noise (Kaplan & Pickett, 1981; Stach, 1990) are evident with the use of two hearing aids as opposed to one. Because one of the most common problems of older users of hearing aids is difficulty in noisy environments, the recommendation for two hearing aids is warranted. The issue of cost is often a deterrent for elderly patients. Because binaural fittings provide important advantages, the audiologist should always recommend two hearing aids if the hearing loss warrants them.

In addition to enhancement of speech perception in noise and localization skills, another strong argument for the use of binaural amplification is the phenomenon of auditory deprivation (Silman et al, 1984). When a person with a bilateral symmetric hearing loss uses a monaural hearing aid, a decline in suprathreshold speech recognition abilities without an accompanying decline in pure-tone or speech thresholds can occur in the ear in which an aid is not worn (Hurley, 1991, 1993; Moore, 1993; Silman, 1994; Silman et al, 1984; 1992). Moore (1993) suggested that an interaural asymmetry occurs when a person uses a monaural hearing aid, causing a decline in the speech recognition abilities of the ear on which an aid is not worn. Auditory deprivation has been documented as occurring as early as 3 months after fitting of monaural amplification (Gatehouse, 1992) and as late as 12 years after the hearing-aid fitting. Silman et al (1992) reported that the average time of onset of evidence of auditory deprivation in adults is 4 years after fitting. Fortunately, in many patients, this phenomenon has been found to be reversible. Silverman and Silman (1990) and Hurley (1991) reported on several patients in whom speech recognition improved in the ear with auditory deprivation after use of binaural hearing aids was begun.

Jerger et al (1993), on the other hand, described the treatment of four elderly patients with binaural interference. These patients had poorer speech recognition scores for binaural than for monaural stimulation. The asymmetry in their speech perception abilities may have been so great that the auditory deprivation effect could not have been reversed. Because of possible auditory deprivation and binaural interference, Jerger (1994) recommended that binaural amplification be used initially for all bilateral hearing losses. If an aid is used in only one ear, a decrease in speech perception ability can be expected in the other ear. This decrease in perception may be reversible if binaural amplification is initiated soon enough.

HEARING-AID BURDEN

Even when patients can perceive benefits from hearing aids, they often still reject using them. The everyday use and upkeep of hearing aids can be overwhelming for some older adults. Changing the battery, inserting the aid, and adjusting the volume can be burdensome tasks to some older users.

The manipulation skills of users of hearing aids need to be considered in the selection of hearing aids. Upfold et al (1990) randomly assigned 244 elderly people with hearing losses to the use of three different types of hearing aids: behind-the-ear (BTE), in-the-ear (ITE), and in-the-canal (ITC). Eight manipulation skills of the users of hearing aids were rated several times—once at the time of fitting and once after each of two or three instruction sessions spaced over several weeks. Users were rated on these factors: aid and mold removal, aid and mold insertion and placement, battery removal, battery replacement, turning on the aid, turning off the aid, volume adjustment, and telecoil selection when applicable. The ITE aid was the easiest to turn on and off and to insert and remove. The subjects found the BTE aid most difficult to insert. The volume control was the most difficult to adjust on the ITC aid. The telecoil switch was easier to learn on the ITE aid than on the BTE aid. Although most of the users learned to manipulate their hearing aids, a few still had difficulty after three instruction sessions, four rating sessions, and practice at home. Women had more difficulty than men inserting the aids. Results of this study showed that 6 percent of elderly patients fit with BTE or ITC aids would stop using the devices because of lack of manipulation skills; only 3 percent of those fit with ITE aids would stop using the aids. The difficulty found with telecoil switches is not uncommon among the elderly population. For some patients who have problems adjusting and manipulating their hearing aids, the audiologist may want to reconsider placing a telecoil option on a hearing aid. These patients may be better served by telephone amplifiers and assistive listening devices other than those that require inductive coupling (see Chapter 6).

To avoid some of the manipulation burdens of hearing aids, audiologists can order special features such as raised volume controls and extraction handles or notches. Another possibility is the use of a remote control for the manipulation of volume, telecoil, and frequency response (Wolf & Powers, 1986). This strategy, however, can be deemed a burden to some patients who do not want to be bothered with extra controls. Careful attention to each patient's needs is necessary to select appropriate manipulation options.

Many improvements in programmable hearing aids offer users more than one frequency response to suit different listening situations. If the patient is having difficulty with standard hearing-aid controls these added frequency responses can become overwhelming. Often it is best to use only one response option for these patients.

OUTCOME MEASUREMENTS

Standard evaluation of the electroacoustic characteristics of a hearing aid should be made at the time of the fitting. Real-ear testing of the insertion gain and outputs should be completed to assure the patient's hearing aids are producing the appropriate amplification for the hearing loss. Functional gain measurements also may be used.

Beyond these physical measurements, the benefits of the use of a hearing aid can be measured with a number of functional assessments. Various self-assessment measurements used by researchers to measure hearing-aid benefits are listed in Table 3–1. In addition to self-perception scales, Cox and Alexander (1991) used their Connected Speech Test to evaluate the benefits of amplification in various environments. This speech perception test has the advantage of using connected speech, which provides contextual cues, and of video disk presentation, which enables the user to ascertain visual cues.

When fitting programmable aids, the audiologist should encourage on-going feedback from the patient by using various taped background noises. After the initial programming, we send patients to a noisy public place so they can assess their comfort with the aids. They then return for small adjustments. During the follow-up visit the next week, additional adjustments are made. During the first weeks of hearing-aid use, we recommend that patients keep a diary of their experiences with the hearing aids. This is helpful in making modifications in both conventional and programmable hearing aids. For example, a slightly uncomfortable mold can be buffed down for comfort. A seemingly small modification might mean the difference between an aid in an ear and an aid in a dresser drawer.

TABLE 3–1 Self-Perception Assessment of the Benefit of Hearing-Aid Use

Research Study	Assessment Used
Golabek et al (1988)	Open-ended questionnaire
Fino et al (1992)	Hearing Handicap Inventory for the Elderly
Newman et al (1991)	Hearing Handicap Inventory for the Elderly—Screening Version
Brooks (1990)	Hearing Aid Review
Cox et al (1991)	Profile of Hearing Aid Performance
Kricos et al (1987)	Hearing Aid Performance Inventory

PERSONAL ADJUSTMENT COUNSELING

The importance of counseling the patient before, during, and after hearing-aid fitting cannot be overemphasized. Clinicians who work with patients with hearing losses can measure the speech-perception benefits of hearing aids using methods of testing in quiet and noise. Self-assessment inventories also provide useful and necessary information on the patient's perceived handicap. One of the best means of choosing the appropriate options and modifications for the hearing aids is to talk to the person with the hearing loss and his or her significant others. Written questionnaires can be helpful, but the audiologist needs to be aware of the patient's ability to read and complete the forms. Because of the high prevalence of visual disorders among the elderly, all forms need to be printed in large type. Kelly and Kahn (1991) evaluated the readability of clinic forms used in various audiologic facilities in the United States and Canada. The results revealed that 39 percent of the forms patients were asked to complete to provide their history were written at the literacy level of university students, 23 percent were at the high school level, 19 percent at the junior high school level, and only 17 percent at the grade school level. Legal documents had even higher readability requirements. It has been estimated that between 17 and 28 million American adults have severely limited reading skills (Laubach Literacy International, 1989). These people would not be able to complete forms without help. Therefore, clinicians who rely solely on written history forms and handicap scales may not be obtaining accurate information. To avoid this problem, handicap scales and histories should be administered verbally whenever possible.

Appropriate expectations of the benefits of hearing-aid use are imperative for successful hearing fit. Patients need to realize that the devices are *aids* to hearing not hearing restorers. Many of the myths about hearing aids must be dispelled. Patients need to understand that they will experience an adjustment period after the fitting. Explaining the typical benefits people experience with hearing aids is helpful. Golabek et al (1988) administered an oral questionnaire on the benefits of amplification to 169 adult users of hearing aids. The environments in which the users reported the most benefit were conversations at home (78.7 percent); listening to television and radio (75.1 percent); conversations at work (43.2 percent); meetings (42.6 percent); shopping (38.5 percent); traffic (33.1 percent); church (29.0 percent); and conversation on the street (24.3 percent). Potential users of hearing aids need to be aware that hearing aids provide the most benefit in favorable listening situations (Cox & Alexander, 1991).

When explaining the various types and options available during the hearing-aid evaluation, the audiologist should have models of the aids available. By observing the patient's manipulation abilities when handling the aids, an audiologist can tell if modifications are needed for volume controls, battery compartments, or other aspects of the aid. If all other factors are equal, an ITE hearing aid is preferable, because it is easiest to insert (Upfold et al, 1990).

At the time of the hearing-aid fitting, the patient needs to be counseled on the benefits and limitations of hearing aids. The client should then be fit with the hearing aids and evaluated with both subjective and objective measures, such as insertion gain. The patient must then be taught the mechanics of the hearing aid. Practice inserting and removing the hearing aids is provided along with instruction on the various controls. Instruction in and an opportunity to practice battery removal and insertion are also provided at this time.

All patients should be encouraged to attend a group hearing-aid adjustment program along with their significant other. My associate and I host a weekly program in our clinic that consists of four different sessions (Holmes & Kemker, 1993). Patients may start at any time. The topics are hearing loss and hearing aids; environmental factors; assistive listening devices; and communication strategies. The cost of the program is included in the cost of the hearing aid. The cost effectiveness of such a program is evidenced by fewer hearing-aid returns, fewer walk-in problems, and patient referrals from participants. A model hearing-aid orientation program for older adults is described in Chapter 9.

FAMILY COUNSELING

Whenever possible, family members and significant others should be included in the counseling process. Hearing impairment affects not only the people with the losses but also those around them (Hetu & Getty, 1991). It causes loss in communication for all those involved, therefore significant others need assistance in dealing with the loss and understanding the benefits and limitations of amplification. As stated earlier, the attitudes of others greatly affect the acceptance of hearing aids. The importance of controlling the environment and giving visual cues along with the use of the hearing aids needs to be emphasized to all involved.

One method of demonstrating the effect of hearing loss to significant others who have normal hearing is to use hearing-loss simulation. Commercial recordings are available that simulate hearing loss with filtered speech with and without noise background. These recordings help with a general understanding of the effects of a high-frequency loss. A better means of demonstrating loss is to use a hearing-loss simulator (HELOS). The HELOS, designed by Erber (1984), is a device that enables the audiologist to simulate hearing loss to significant others through the use of audio or video tape played through a simulator. The HELOS provides frequency shaping of the signal and some distortion characteristics. Perceptual difficulties similar to those demonstrated by people with hearing losses have been demonstrated by normal hearing listeners using the HELOS (Gagne & Erber, 1987). By using video tape simulations, the significant other is able to experience the advantages of using visual cues. The hearing aid can also be routed though the system to show some of its benefits and limitations.

CARE AND MAINTENANCE OF A HEARING AID

Careful instruction in the care and maintenance of a hearing aid is beneficial for both the patient and the clinician. Fewer returns and walk-in problems occur in an office when users of hearing aids are made aware of simple maintenance techniques.

In our clinic, each user of a hearing aid is given a list of the tools necessary for proper upkeep of their hearing aids: wax pick, hearing-aid dehumidifier or drying kit, soft toothbrush, and extra batteries. The wax pick and hearing-aid dehumidifier are dispensed with the hearing aid. We have found that for older patients a toothbrush to clean the microphone and receiver opening is easier to manipulate than the small brush that usually is provided by the manufacturer. In humid climates such as Florida the use of a drying kit can extend the life of a hearing aid. Attention to proper use of the drying agent is needed. One elderly patient returned to our clinic with two melted hearing aids after he placed both the drying kit and hearing aids in the oven.

The tools are demonstrated and the patient is required to demonstrate his or her ability to clean the hearing aids. Written instructions on the care and maintenance of the aids are given to each user. Instructions specific to each patient's aids are also given, such as how to remove or clean the wax guards. Family members or significant others should be present if possible, so they are able to help the user if necessary.

INSTRUCTIONS FOR THE CARE AND CLEANING OF HEARING AIDS

1. Keep the hearing aid dry. Protect it from rain, remove it before taking a bath or shower, do not swim while wearing the aid.
2. Remove or cover your hearing aid when applying hair spray.
3. Always carry a spare battery.
4. Store hearing aids and batteries in a safe place when not in use. Batteries and hearing aids can be ingested by small children or pets.
5. Wipe off the aid with a tissue or dry cloth whenever you remove it from your ear.
6. Store your aid in a hearing-aid dehumidifier every night.
7. Remove the battery when aid is not in use.
8. Perform the following procedures each morning:
   - Check opening for wax.
   - Brush hearing-aid microphone and receiver with toothbrush. Make sure to hold hearing aid so dirt and wax can fall out easily while brushing it.
   - If needed, clean opening with wax pick.
   - Disconnect the earmold and clean the tubing with a pipe cleaner if necessary (for behind-the-ear aids).
9. Disconnect and wash the earmold, if necessary. Do not use alcohol on the earmold. *Make sure the earmold is totally dry before reconnecting it to the hearing aid* (for behind-the-ear aids).

Most manufacturers provide the consumer with printed information on the workings of the hearing aid, controls, and maintenance. The concerns about the readability of these materials are the same as for clinic forms (Kelly, 1993). In evaluating the readability of 109 documents obtained from 23 hearing-aid companies, Kelly classified 57.7 percent at the university level, 22 percent at the high school level, 15.6 percent at the junior high level, and 6.4 percent at the grade school level. Even the diagrams in most brochures can be confusing to the average consumer. Technical terms must be explained to users of hearing aids in appropriate language. Figure 3–1 shows hearing diagrams similar to those found in many information flyers. Note the use of technical terms and the cluttered appearance. Figure 3–2 illustrates diagrams that have been redesigned to improve understanding for the typical patient.

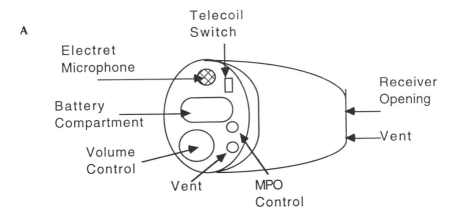

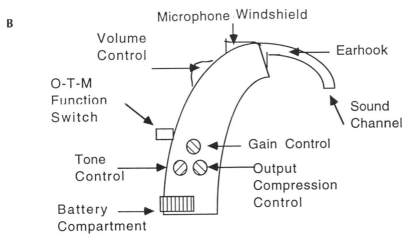

FIGURE 3–1 *Examples of typical hearing-aid diagrams. Typical labeling of (A) in-the-ear hearing aid and (B) behind-the-ear hearing aid, using technical terms.*

(Courtesy of L. Kelly)

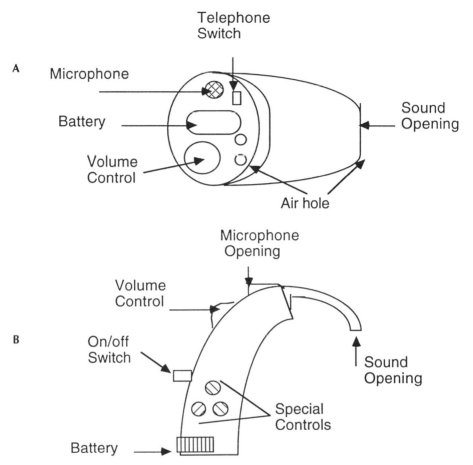

FIGURE 3–2 *Examples of hearing-aid diagrams modified for readability. Improved labeling of (A) in-the-ear hearing aid and (B) behind-the-ear hearing aid using less technical terms.* (Courtesy of L. Kelly)

CONCLUSION

Hearing aids can greatly improve the quality of life of older people with hearing impairments. Appropriate expectations about the benefits and limitations of amplification are necessary for both clients and significant others for the client to accept and adjust to the use of hearing aids. Counseling is extremely important to the entire process of fitting hearing aids on the elderly.

The presence of CAPDs in some of the elderly population with hearing losses provides challenges to fitting these patients with amplification. Advances in hearing-aid technology have lessened some of the difficulties in fitting elderly people, including severe speech perception problems. Audiologists must be aware of the unique problems the elderly often face when using amplification, such as speech perception difficulties and poor manipulation skills. These problems can be overcome, providing patients optimal benefits from the use of hearing aids.

REFERENCES

Bess, F., Lichtenstein, M., & Logan, S. (1990). Audiologic assessment of the hearing-impaired elderly. In W.B. Rintelmann (Ed.), *Hearing assessment* (pp. 511-548). Austin: Pro-Ed.

Bess, F., Logan, S.A., Lichtenstein, M., & Hedley, A. (1987). Early identification and referral of hearing-impaired elderly. In M.S. Robinette & C.D. Bauch (Eds.), *Proceedings of a symposium in audiology* (pp. 1-27). Rochester: Mayo Clinic & Mayo Foundation.

Brooks, D.N. (1985) Factors relating to the under-use of postaural hearing aids. *British Journal of Audiology, 19,* 211-217.

Brooks, D.N. (1989) The effect of attitude on benefit obtained from hearing aids. *British Journal of Audiology 23,* 1-11.

Brooks, D.N. (1990). Measures for the assessment of hearing aid provision and rehabilitation. *British Journal of Audiology, 24,* 229-233.

Byrne, D., & Dillon, H. (1986). The National Acoustic Laboratories' (NAL) new procedure for selecting the gain and frequency response of a hearing aid. *Ear and Hearing, 7,* 257-265.

Byrne, D., Noble, W., & LePage, B. (1992). Effects of long-term binaural and unilateral fitting of different hearing aid types on the ability to locate sounds. *Journal of the American Academy of Audiology, 3,* 369-382.

Cox, R.M., & Alexander, G.C. (1991). Hearing aid benefit in everyday environments. *Ear and Hearing, 12,* 127-139.

Crandell, C. (1991). Individual speech recognition susceptibility to noise: Implications for hearing aid selection. *Ear and Hearing, 12* (Suppl.), 520-532.

Davis, J.W., & Mueller, H.G. (1987). Hearing aid selection. In H.G. Mueller & V.C. Geoffrey (Eds.), *Communication disorders in aging* (pp. 408-436). Washington: Gallaudet University Press.

Erber, N.P. (1984). Simulation of hearing loss. *Hearing Technology Review, 1,* 6-7.

Fino, M.S., Bess, F., Lichtenstein, M.J., & Logan, S.A. (1992). Factors differentiating elderly hearing aid wearers vs. non-wearers. *Hearing Instruments, 43,* 6-10.

Franks, J.R., & Beckmann N.J. (1985). Rejection of hearing aids: Attitudes of a geriatric sample. *Ear and Hearing, 6,* 161-166.

Gabbard, S.A. (1994). AARP's report on hearing aids. *Audiology Today 6,* 15.

Gallup Organization (1980). A survey concerning hearing problems and hearing aids in the United States. Princeton: Gallup.

Gagné, J.P., & Erber, N.P. (1987). Simulation of sensorineural hearing loss impairment. *Ear and Hearing, 8,* 232-243.

Gatehouse, S. (1992). The timecourse and magnitude of perceptual acclimation to frequency responses: Evidence from monaural fitting of hearing aids. *Journal of the Acoustical Society of America, 92,* 1258-1268.

Golabek, W., Nowakowka, M., Siwiec, H. & Stephens, S.D.G. (1988). Self-reported benefits of hearing aids by the hearing impaired. *British Journal of Audiology, 22,* 183-186.

Gordon-Salant, S. & Sherlock, L.P. (1992). Performance with an adaptive frequency response hearing aid in a sample of elderly hearing-impaired listeners. *Ear and Hearing, 13,* 255-261.

Harless, E.L., & McConnell, F. (1982). Effects of hearing aid use on self concept in older persons. *Journal of Speech and Hearing Disorders, 47,* 305-309.

Hayes, D., & Jerger, J. (1979). Aging and use of hearing aids. *Scandinavian Audiology, 8,* 33-40.

Hetu, R., & Getty, L. (1991). Development of a rehabilitation program for people affected with occupational hearing loss. II. Results from group intervention with 48 workers and their spouses. *Audiology, 30,* 317-329.

Holmes, A.E., & Kemker, F.J. (1993). Beyond the hearing aid fitting. Presented at the American Academy of Audiology Annual Convention, April 15-18, 1993, Phoenix.

Humes, L.E., & Kirn, E.U. (1990). The reliability of functional gain. *Journal of Speech and Hearing Disorders, 55,* 193-197.

Hurley, R.M. (1991). *Hearing aid use and auditory deprivation: A prospective study.* Poster presented at the Annual Convention of the American Academy of Audiology, April 25-28, 1993, Denver.

Hurley, R.M. (1993). Monaural hearing aid effect: Case presentation. *Journal of the American Academy of Audiology, 4,* 285-295.

Iler, K., Danhauer, J., & Mulac, A. (1982). Peer perceptions of geriatrics wearing hearing aids. *Journal of Speech and Hearing Disorders, 47,* 433-438.

Jerger, J. (1994). The phenomenon of binaural interference. *Hearing Instruments, 45,* 29.

Jerger, J., Lew, H.L., Silman, S., & Chmiel R. (1993). Case studies in binaural interference: Converging evidence from behavioral and electrophysiologic measures. *Journal of the American Academy of Audiology, 4,* 122-131.

Johnson, C., Danhauer, J., & Edwards, R. (1982). The "hearing aid effect" in geriatrics: Fact or fiction? *Hearing Instruments, 33,* 10-24.

Kaplan, H., & Pickett, J.M. (1981). Effects of dichotic/diotic versus monotic presentation on speech understanding in noise in elderly hearing-impaired listeners. *Ear and Hearing, 2,* 202-207.

Kelly, L.J. (1993). The readability of hearing aid brochures. Presented at the Academy of Rehabilitative Audiology Summer Institute, June 10-13, 1993, Howey-in-the-Hills, Fla.

Kelly, L.J., & Kahn, A. (1991). Illiteracy and hearing loss management: The readability of clinic forms. *Journal of the Academy of Rehabilitative Audiology, 24,* 35-42.

Kricos, P.B., Lesner, S.A., & Sandridge, S.A. (1991). Expectations of older adults regarding the use of hearing aids. *Journal of the American Academy of Audiology, 2,* 129-133.

Kricos, P.B., Lesner, S.A., Sandridge, S.A., & Yanke, R.B. (1987). Perceived benefits of amplification as a function of central auditory status in the elderly. *Ear and Hearing, 8,* 337-342.

Laubach Literacy International (1989). *Tutor handbook.* Syracuse: New Reader's Press.

Leijon, A., Eriksson-Mangold, M., & Bech-Karlsen, A. (1984). Preferred hearing aid gain and bass-cut in relation to prescriptive fitting. *Scandinavian Audiology, 13,* 157-162.

Malinoff, R.L., & Weinstein, B.E. (1989). Measurements of hearing aid benefit in the elderly. *Ear and Hearing, 10,* 354-360.

Moore, D.R. (1993). Plasticity of binaural hearing and some possible mechanisms following late-onset deprivation. *Journal of the American Academy of Audiology, 4,* 277-283.

Mulrow, C.D., Aguilar, C., Endicott, J.E., et al (1990). Quality-of-life changes and hearing impairment: A randomized trial. *Annals of Internal Medicine, 113,* 188-194.

Mulrow, C.D., Tuley, M.R., & Aguilar, C. (1992). Correlates of successful hearing aid use in older adults. *Ear and Hearing, 13,* 108-113.

Newman, C.W., Jacobson, G.P., Hug, G.A., Weinstein, B.E., & Malinoff, R.L. (1991). Practical method for quantifying hearing aid benefit in older adults. *Journal of the American Academy of Audiology, 2,* 70-75.

Parving, A., & Phillip, B. (1991). Use and benefit of hearing aids in the tenth decade—and beyond. *Audiology, 30,* 61-69.

Ryals, B.M., & Auther, L.L. (1990). Differences in hearing instrument gain as a function of age. *Hearing Instruments, 41,* 26-28.

Schow, R.L. (1982). Success of hearing aid fittings in nursing homes. *Ear and Hearing, 3,* 173-177.

Shadden, B.B., & Raiford, C.A. (1984). Factors influencing service utilization by older individuals. *Journal of Communication Disorders, 17,* 209-224.

Silman, S. (1994). Auditory deprivation: Are two aided ears better than one? *Hearing Instruments, 45,* 28-29.

Silman, S., Gelfand, S.A., & Silverman, C.A. (1984). Effects of monaural versus binaural hearing aids. *Journal of the Acoustical Society of America, 76,* 1357-1362.

Silman, S., Silverman, C.A., Emmer, M.B., & Gelfand, S.A. (1992). Adult-onset auditory deprivation. *Journal of the American Academy of Audiology, 3,* 390-396.

Silverman, C.A., & Silman, S. (1990). Apparent auditory deprivation from monaural amplification and recovery with binaural amplification. *Journal of the American Academy of Audiology, 1,* 175-180.

Smedley, T.C., & Schow, R.L. (1994). Frustrations with hearing aid use: Candid observations from the elderly. *Hearing Instruments, 43,* 21-27.

Stach, B.A. (1990). Hearing aid amplification and central processing disorders. In R.E. Sandlin (Ed.), *Handbook of hearing aid amplification: Vol II. Clinical considerations and fitting practices* (pp. 87-111). Austin: Pro-Ed.

Stach, B.A., Spretnejak, M.L., & Jerger, J.F. (1990). The prevalence of central presbycusis in a clinical population. *Journal of the American Academy of Audiology, 1,* 109-115.

Taylor, K.S. (1993). Self-perceived and audiometric evaluations of hearing aid benefit in the elderly. *Ear and Hearing, 14,* 390-394.

Thibodeau, L.M., & Schmitt, L. (1988). A report on condition of hearing aids in nursing homes and retirement centers. *Journal of the Academy of Rehabilitative Audiology, 21,* 113-119.

Upfold, L.J., May, A.E., & Battaglia, J.A. (1990). Hearing aid manipulation skills in the elderly population: A comparison of ITE, BTE, and ITC aids. *British Journal of Audiology, 24,* 311-318.

Ventry, I., & Weinstein, B. (1983). Identification of elderly people with hearing problems. *ASHA, 7,* 37-42.

Wolf, H.P., & Powers, T.A. (1986). Remote control: The invisible touch. *Hearing Journal, 39,* 10, 18-20.

Chapter 4

Effective and Relevant Programming

Judy Abrahamson

Successful fitting of amplification is not the appropriate end point of hearing care for all clients. This is especially true for older adults. Lieberth (1992) stated that

> the primary determinant of the success of programs lies in the belief by audiologist, hearing-impaired adult, their families, and the public in general that aural rehabilitation may be a necessary, albeit short-term component of a comprehensive program of hearing health care for some hearing-impaired persons and that it can improve the communication abilities of those persons who take advantage of it (p. 38).

This chapter describes the components of audiologic rehabilitation and provides an overview of factors the practitioner must consider in planning programs. Suggestions are made about materials for use in remediation.

GOALS FOR THE AUDIOLOGIC REMEDIATION PROCESS

Montgomery (1991) formulated five goals for adult audiologic rehabilitation.

Goals for Adult Audiologic Rehabilitation
1. Maximizing sensory input involves supplying the best possible visual and amplified auditory signal
2. Maximizing sensory (auditory and visual) integration involves making the best use of amplification and audiovisual perception of speech
3. Maximizing cognitive processing involves applying past experience, knowledge of the current situation, and language to improving recognition of incomplete sensory messages
4. Maximizing family and work communication involves addressing specific work and home environments
5. Maximizing interactive communication involves developing an assertive and interactive way of communicating and repairing breakdowns

The term *older adults* describes people with a dramatic range of abilities and needs. Establishing appropriate goals for audiologic rehabilitation therefore requires careful attention to individual differences. Hearing status; use of amplification; visual, motor, and cognitive ability; living and working environments; the presence or ability of significant others to take part in the rehabilitation process; social and vocational demands for communication; and health status are a few of the factors that must be understood before appropriate goals may be selected.

Behaviorally defined goals make it easier for the clinician to select appropriate techniques and strategies for effecting change and to identify and monitor progress. Clearly stated goals are an essential part of treatment plans and are an essential component of the documentation required for third-party payment.

A behaviorally stated goal should specify who, what, where, when, and how much? Outcome goals should clearly specify the behavior to be changed, identify who will perform the behavior, indicate the conditions under which the targeted behavior will occur, specify the date on which the goal will be reached, and include a realistic rate of occurrence of the behavior necessary to meet the goal. Roberts and Bryant (1992) provided a comprehensive review of goal setting for rehabilitative audiology as a continuation of the diagnostic process. They stated that "goal-setting should be viewed as a flexible process, subject to modification and refinement" (p. 82). They suggested that active client involvement in selecting and carefully stating goals is important for several reasons. It motivates clients to develop and maintain new behaviors and decreases the risk of failure; it allows clients to rehearse new behaviors as they interact with their environment; and it gives clients a framework for evaluating their progress.

The type of intervention (individual or group) can influence the goals that are developed. Goals for individual participants in a group can differ somewhat, but they are usually less specific than is possible for individual intervention. Such goals may be demonstrating improved knowledge of information presented in a class. In counseling groups, specific individualized goals are usually not possible. Adjustment to the hearing loss or attitude and behavior changes are frequently an important component of the intervention, but these qualities are difficult to describe much less quantify. General goals of group counseling focus on educating members about coping strategies, behaviors, or factors that influence communication.

The following is a list of examples of goals that may be appropriate for older adults in a variety of settings.

- The number of times Mrs. Smith moves to the same room as her husband to initiate conversation will increase by 40 percent over baseline within the next 4 months. Mr. Smith has measured baseline occurrence of this behavior to be one instance during a 4-hour period on a weekday afternoon. He will continue to monitor this behavior on a monthly basis.

- Within 2 months, Mrs. Lee's rate for audiovisual speech tracking with a signal-to-noise ratio (S/N) of +5 dB will increase by 20 percent over her baseline of 18 words per minute.
- Mr. Jones will score 80 percent on the test of hearing-aid care and maintenance developed at his center after he completes the hearing-aid orientation class. His pretest score was 28 percent.
- Mr. Lopez will verbalize an understanding of the benefits of informing others of his hearing loss and making specific requests for clarification during the last group meeting.
- When shown a floor plan and photograph of a restaurant 1 month after completion of class, Mrs. Jones will identify three environmental factors that may interfere with her husband's communication and will make four suggestions of strategies she can use to improve their conversational fluency in that setting. On pretest, she identified one noise source as a potential problem but made no suggestions for improvement.

CONSIDERATIONS IN THE REMEDIATION PROCESS

Trust Relationship

The clinician must have state-of-the-art knowledge and skills related to amplification, assistive technology, audiologic rehabilitation evaluation, and rehabilitative treatment procedures. Expertise, however, is not sufficient to ensure success. A trust relationship between client and clinician is necessary for client change to occur (Schum, 1993). Roberts and Bryant (1992) described goals for clinicians that involve establishing this relationship and producing conditions conducive to client change: "The clinician must actively sense and communicate empathy, genuineness, and unconditional positive regard" (p. 82). Luterman (1991) also emphasized trust. He stated that "unfortunately, many professional relationships are not built on trust, and there can be no growth in relationships unless trust is present" (Luterman, 1991, p. 37). He suggested that trust is built by three basic elements: (1) caring is conveyed to the client by active, sensitive, and nonjudgmental listening; (2) consistency involves treating clients as reliable individuals (eg, starting and ending therapy sessions on time and apologizing for and correcting errors); (3) credibility is earned over time by what the practitioner knows and the manner in which he or she conveys this information. Saying "I don't know" can strengthen, rather than harm, credibility.

Physical Environment

Room Requirements

Individual therapy can be conducted in a variety of settings. A quiet room with adequate lighting and comfortable seating is required. In retirement centers and nursing homes, it is often appropriate to conduct some sessions in dayrooms, dining rooms, or bedrooms. It is best to use these more difficult settings only after initial success has been achieved in a quiet therapy room. Practitioners in the field know from experience that ideal settings are not always available. Creativity is often required to ensure that a private setting is provided and that activities are appropriate for the noise levels and distractions present.

Group therapy is best conducted in a room that allows comfortable seating for all participants around a table (preferably round) to allow for optimal ease of speechreading and to promote peer interaction. A circle of chairs is adequate if written material is not distributed to group members. Some isolation from busy areas within a facility is desirable for two reasons. First, the room is likely to be more quiet, and second, when a sound system is used, other people in the building are less likely to overhear and be disturbed by the group.

Flexibility in therapy rooms is desirable but not always possible. Lighting should be adequate for speechreading. If video tapes are used, ability to dim the lights is helpful. Adjustable lighting and movable furniture can be useful in teaching clients to manipulate their communication environment. Open blinds that cause a glare can be used, for example, to encourage a client to request a seating change or to close the blinds. Noise sources or awkward viewing angles also can be useful in providing opportunities to practice environmental management. External noise sources and visual distractions, however, should be absent because many activities require ideal listening and viewing conditions, at least during the initial stages of therapy.

Audiovisual Equipment

The use of personal amplification is a prerequisite for auditory rehabilitation, except for the rare instance when amplification is not recommended. A sound system that can be used with or without personal amplification is helpful with groups, but is not essential. Abrahamson (1991) found a system composed of an audio loop, a speaker, an amplifier, and two microphones to be practical. The practitioner wears a lapel microphone, and a second microphone, passed from speaker to speaker, has two functions. It ensures a favorable S/N that allows clients with severe hearing losses to successfully follow group discussions. It is also useful in maintaining order by allowing only one person to speak at a time.

Audio tape recordings of sessions allow the clinician to count verbal communication behaviors as a means of documenting improvement. Tape recorders can be the source of competing background noise. A sound level meter is also needed if auditory or audiovisual training is to be performed at various S/Ns.

Video recorders and monitors, when available, can serve a wide variety of functions. In addition to being useful for instruction, video recordings of interactions allow clients to observe and evaluate their own behaviors in role-playing or other activities. Some evaluation procedures, such as TOPICON (Erber, 1988), require analysis of videotaped conversations.

Materials

Practitioners in clinical settings may feel some apprehension about initiating long-term rehabilitation programs in conjunction with hearing-aid fittings. Developing appropriate materials may seem to be a daunting addition to an already busy clinical schedule. Commercially available materials can make this task manageable. Photographs, objects, or special material such as QUEST?AR (Erber, 1988) can be used as stimuli in conversational fluency training. Written passages of interest to the client at the appropriate reading level are required for speech tracking activities. Materials that can be used for rehabilitative activities are described in this section. Considerations for developing and selecting materials to meet different therapeutic needs are also discussed.

Written Materials

The clinician has a variety of written materials from which to choose. Some can be used as therapeutic materials for auditory training, speechreading, strategies training, or assertiveness training activities (see Chapter 10), and others are appropriate for home study. A lending library of educational books written for clients and family members can be useful. Other materials can be used for in-service training of related professionals.

Literacy should be considered when choosing commercially available materials or developing new written materials for older adults. Kelly (1993) examined educational materials prepared by manufacturers of hearing aids. She found that 58 percent of these materials were written at a 12th grade reading level, the level recommended for technical writing. A fifth or sixth grade reading level seems appropriate for older adults with hearing impairments. This level is considered functionally literate and is the average reading level of most newspapers. Computer programs are available with which the clinician can determine the reading levels of texts.

Because visual deficits are common among the older population, type size should be considered. Fourteen-point type is appropriate for general use, although some people may need larger print. The visual contrast of print materials should be considered. A creative clinician may choose brightly colored paper for aesthetic reasons, not realizing that the lack of contrast between print and paper may cause problems for some clients. With the advent of personal computers and desktop publishing, a clinician who develops his or her written materials can customize them to meet the needs of individual clients.

Audiovisual Materials

Commercially prepared audio cassettes are available on a range of educational topics, but their use is limited to clients with good speech recognition ability. For example, AUDITEC of St. Louis (1981) has produced a set of auditory training tapes with accompanying response sheets that can be used by some clients as home study materials. Video tapes are available that can be used to educate (Compton, 1991), stimulate class discussion (Trychin, 1987), and to provide individual practice (Greenwald, 1984).

Examples of materials that can be useful for different components of an audiologic rehabilitative program are included in the discussion of training components later in this chapter. Nonexhaustive lists of commercially available materials and references are provided in Appendixes 4–1 and 4–2.

Service Delivery Models and Scheduling

Questions related to service delivery models have a direct effect on scheduling. Several of these questions are addressed separately as they relate to audiologic rehabilitation.

Where Should Therapy Be Conducted?

Should therapy be conducted in a clinic, in a community setting, or in the client's residence? The clinic is usually most convenient for the clinician. Alpiner (1982) suggested community-based programs as a more effective means to reach people in need of services. Many services are now provided in nursing homes. Because older adults are more likely to have transportation problems than younger ones, services provided in the residence or retirement home may be more accessible.

When Should Treatment Be Given?

Therapy for older adults with hearing impairments should generally be provided during traditional working hours. If treatment is offered at a retirement community, early evening sessions are possible. As a rule, the senior population tends to be less likely than a younger population to drive or take part in activities at night.

How Frequently Should Treatment Be Given?

Flexibility in scheduling individual clients is important. Decisions are influenced by time constraints of the clinician and the client, availability of facilities, and clients' health or mobility. Daily half-hour sessions with a nursing-home resident may be appropriate, whereas hour-long weekly meetings with an active retiree may be all that is possible. As therapy progresses and the client's goals focus on generalizing skills to situations outside therapy, the frequency of sessions may decrease.

How Long Should Each Therapy Session Last?

A client's stamina and attention span as well as the therapy activities should influence this decision. Fifteen minutes of speech tracking in noise or analytic speechreading activities can be tiring, whereas a lively group discussion that lasts 60 minutes may not be. Activities that require intense auditory and visual concentration should be interspersed with less demanding activities. Rest periods are necessary for clients to participate in therapeutic activities at their maximum performance. If sessions last more than 45 minutes, breaks should be given.

Should Therapy Be Conducted Individually or in Groups?

Many activities described later in this chapter require individual treatment. Lesner (1992), however, stated that groups provide the most cost-effective and practical means of providing audiologic rehabilitative services to older adults (see Chapter 9 for a model group program).

When Should Rehabilitation Services End?

Discharge planning is relatively straightforward in individual therapy. The American Speech-Language-Hearing Association (ASHA) (1993) specified that goals and objectives should be reviewed periodically and that dismissal or discharge planning should occur continually throughout treatment. Analogous decisions about groups are not as straightforward.

How Long Should a Group Meet?

The answer to this question depends on the function of the group. Two types of audiologic rehabilitation groups can be found: instructional and interactive. Instructional classes, such as speechreading or hearing-aid orientation classes, should meet long enough to cover the required material. Feeham, Samuelson, and Seymour (1982) described a series of 14 speechreading lessons. Wayner (1990a,b) provided materials for three classes after hearing-aid fitting. Lesner and Kricos (1991) described a model hearing-aid orientation program that spans 5 weeks and involves both clients with hearing impairments and their significant others (see Chapter 9).

Alpiner (1982) described interactive groups as using a progressive approach with a counseling-type rather than an instructional method. An example of an interactive group is found in Abrahamson (1991). Because peer interaction is essential in this approach, the same group of people should meet for an extended period of time.

Hearing care clinicians must consider the foregoing questions as they attempt to address the needs of their clients. Scheduling individual and group therapy requires commitment and creativity. Although the planning time required for audiologic rehabilitation varies among activities, clinicians should allow preparation time in their schedules. This time decreases as the clinician becomes familiar with the activities and develops a library of easily accessible and modifiable materials.

CHARACTERISTICS OF SUCCESSFUL PROGRAMS

A successful audiologic rehabilitation program is one in which the communication ability of the client improves. A successful program requires a successful clinician, a successful client, appropriate goals and activities, and a philosophical and theoretic framework in which to view the process. These components are discussed separately.

Successful Clinicians

The following characteristics can be said to describe a successful clinician who works with older adults with hearing impairments.

- Ability to develop a trust relationship with clients and family
- Motivation to provide audiologic rehabilitation
- Realization that hearing-aid fitting is the first step and not usually the only step in audiologic rehabilitation
- Belief that audiologic rehabilitation is a worthwhile professional activity and charges accordingly
- Ability to determine when hearing-aid fitting is not sufficient to meet clients' communication needs
- Awareness of the physical and mental changes that exist with hearing loss in older adults and ability to modify evaluation and treatment procedures in ways that meet the needs of the individual client
- Ability to persuade administrators to invest resources of time and materials in rehabilitation services
- Ability to guide clients in goal-setting process
- Ability to modify materials and oral presentation style to meet the needs of clients
- Ability to present information in a manner that is understandable and motivating to the client
- Ability to modify interaction with clients to reflect awareness of cultural diversity in reactions to acquired hearing loss
- Willingness to establish long-term relationships with clients
- Willingness and ability to provide auditory rehabilitation evaluation
- Willingness to modify personal appearance to reduce distractions during therapy (mustaches trimmed, earrings small and non-dangling, clothing of neutral solid color or small pattern)

- Ability to conduct history interview in such a way that functional communication needs are addressed and initial rehabilitation goal formulation begins
- Ability to modify activities in groups to ensure that all participants are given practice items at appropriately challenging levels of difficulty

Successful Clients

The following characteristics describe successful clients in an auditory rehabilitation program.

- Motivation to attend and learn
- Willingness to participate in class activities
- Willingness to complete homework assignments and practice outside therapy
- Motivation to examine long-standing communication behaviors
- Willingness to try new things
- Willingness to share insights and experiences with others
- Eagerness to learn from peers and interest in the success of other clients
- Willingness to involve family and friends in the process of improving communication
- Willingness to inform communication partners of the hearing loss and the associated needs
- Willingness to be assertive in managing the hearing loss
- Willingness to routinely wear hearing aids and use assistive technology whenever possible
- Willingness to develop new skills or knowledge as the result of participation
- Willingness to develop a sense of advocacy concerning the needs and rights of people with hearing impairments

Successful Individual Programs

Successful programs for individual clients have the following characteristics.

- Motivated clients who are involved in setting appropriate goals
- Evaluations to provide baseline measurements and documentation of progress toward goals
- Activities appropriate for the client's abilities and needs
- Appropriate meeting location and audiovisual equipment
- Spouse, caregiver, or significant other participation in goal setting, when possible

Successful Group Programs

Instructional Groups

Successful instructional groups have the following characteristics.

- General goals for participants related to the instructional content material
- Documentation of individual baseline and post-treatment performance
- Material presented in a manner that is understandable and motivating to clients
- Activities modified to ensure that all participants are given practice items at appropriately challenging levels of difficulty
- Good attendance and retention rates by participants
- Family participation (desirable, but not essential for most instructional classes)
- Improved client skills or knowledge of the clients as a result of participation

Interactive Groups

Successful interactive groups have the following characteristics.

- Clinician (as facilitator) talking no more than 30 percent of the time
- High rate of family participation
- Goals that focus on educating members about coping strategies, behaviors, or factors that influence communication
- Activities that focus on peer interaction
- Activities that facilitate clients' abilities to apply new information and behaviors in their daily lives
- Thorough planning by the clinician

SPEECHREADING TRAINING

Speechreading is the component of audiologic rehabilitation with the most name recognition among the general population. Although *speechreading* is considered a more accurate term, *lipreading* is more commonly understood by clients. These terms are used interchangeably in this chapter. Most people have unrealistic expectations about the potential benefit of lip-reading. For lipreading training to be successful, the client should accept that it is a supplement to and not a substitute for auditory speech recognition. Education about the relative visibility of speech sounds, the homophenous (look-alike) nature of many speech sounds, speed of articulation, and variations between individual speakers' mouth movements, speech patterns, and dialect can help develop realistic expectations. Cherry and Rubenstein (1988) suggested that most adults with acquired hearing losses have developed some speechreading skills, but would benefit from learning to improve their use of the visual cues of speech.

Johnson and Caccamise (1982) emphasized the need for visual assessment before training begins. Visual problems become more common as age increases (United States National Health Survey, 1968). Changes in visual abilities associated with aging are described in Chapter 1. These changes can affect the success of lipreading programs. There is evidence that lipreading ability decreases with age even when visual acuity is constant (Pelson & Prather, 1974). Clinicians should make sure that clients wear their corrective lenses during therapy and that correct viewing distance is understood and used by the client.

Suggested Activities

The aim of analytic activities is to develop perceptual proficiency. Groups of speech sounds are visually similar, such as /p/, /b/, and /m/. These groups of sounds that look the same are called visemes. Sounds formed by the lips are easier to see than those formed by the back of the tongue. Viseme groups can be presented in order of increasing visual difficulty. The specific movements of each can be demonstrated. In visually contrasting word pairs, sounds within viseme groups are compared with sounds from other viseme groups. Words in sentences are used to demonstrate that context must be used to determine if a visual stimulus is *bear*, *pear*, or *mare*, for example. The quick recognition and identification exercises described by Jeffers and Barley (1976) address improving perceptual skills, visual memory, and speed of visual perception. For recognition, sets of words that differ by one viseme are printed on a board and then presented visually by the instructor in varied order. The client is asked to repeat the words in the same order as the instructor. For identification, the instructor presents a word and the client identifies it and suggests reasonable visual alternatives. For example, the client may identify the word *pill* and suggest that *mill* looks the same. These suggestions are written on the board and presented in sentences.

Synthetic activities involve teaching the person to use situational and topical clues to aid in speechreading connected discourse, to be flexible in the identification of messages, and to learn to confirm message accuracy (Perry, 1977). Ordman and Ralli (1976) provided related sentences to train clients to use vocabulary from one sentence as an aid in understanding other sentences on the same topic. Jeffers and Barley (1976) included training in association to improve perceptual closure, conceptual closure, and flexibility. Key words can be written and used to provide a context for one of several sentences. Longer material, such as paragraphs or short stories, can discourage the tendency to try to understand every word and to focus on receiving the main idea of an utterance. Newspaper clippings or short stories brought by clients make excellent material for synthetic exercises. Appendixes 4–1 and 4–2 contain a summary of materials that are available for all aspects of audiologic rehabilitation, including lipreading training, for older adults. Chapter 10 also contains a variety of materials to be used in lipreading, auditory, and audiovisual training.

Montgomery (1984) suggested that poor viewing strategies used by patients can interfere with speechreading or prevent them from performing at their perceptual potential. Clients may not watch the speaker's face consistently. Looking around, turning one's better ear to the speaker, and looking at the speaker's eyes are examples of poor viewing strategies. Patients should be taught to focus on the speaker's face to lipread at their best. Environmental cues can be obtained through peripheral vision or during pauses in the conversation.

Tracking

De Filippo and Scott (1978) developed a procedure for training and evaluating the reception of continuous discourse. This procedure was developed for work with vibrotactile aids, but its use quickly spread to speechreading, auditory training, and audiovisual training purposes. The sender reads phrase by phrase from a prepared text. The receiver repeats word for word what was said. If correct repetition does not occur, the sender applies strategies until the receiver can provide a verbatim repetition. The sender and receiver continue this procedure for a specified period of time (5-minute blocks are convenient). The number of words in the text that were repeated verbatim per minute is computed and recorded. Clients can chart their tracking rate in words per minute (wpm) to monitor their progress. This chart can be motivational as well as useful in documenting improvement.

Owens and Telleen (1981) modified the task of speech tracking to focus on communication training and to require the receiver to request specific strategies until he or she can give the verbatim repetition. The clinician can tape sessions and count strategy use as a means of documenting performance. Video taping is preferred because nonverbal strategies such as gestures and watching the mouth can be included, but audio tape can be used as well.

The details of familiarizing clients and conducting the procedure are beyond the scope of this chapter. Reviews are provided by De Filippo (1988) and Owens and Raggio (1987). Although counting the words in passages to compute word-per-minute scores can be tedious, this procedure can be useful. It can be easily modified for auditory training or audiovisual training. Background noise or visual distractions can be added to make tracking more challenging. Chapter 10 provides a variety of passages that can be used for tracking.

AUDIOVISUAL COMMUNICATION TRAINING

In most instances, communication training should focus on audiovisual speech recognition because this is the way most older adults with hearing impairments process everyday conversations. Lipreading alone can be a frustrating task for client and clinician. Because lipreading is a supplement to and not a substitute for hearing, many authors have suggested that audiovisual training is more appropriate than speechreading in the absence of sound (Hardick, 1977; Alpiner, 1982.) The benefit of adding the visual stimulus to auditory speech recognition tasks is well known (Binnie et al, 1974), the effect being more pronounced at low sensation levels.

The lipreading activities described in the previous section can be presented with the addition of auditory information. Adaptive procedures, in which the clinician modifies stimuli in response to the client's success with a previous stimulus, can be used to change viewing angle, increase volume of speech, or add distraction. Both synthetic and analytic tasks lend themselves to audiovisual presentation.

Garstecki (1981) provided a practical framework for training audiovisual speech perception by manipulating the redundancy of the message. The following four parameters of the message are controlled: (1) message types vary from syllables to words, sentences, paragraphs, and stories; (2) competing noise varies from cafeteria and multispeaker babble to quiet; (3) S/Ns vary from +12 dB to -6 dB; (4) situation cues vary from distractions to descriptive cues. The client's baseline performance is measured for monosyllabic words with multitalker babble at a 0-dB S/N with no distractions. Each of the four parameters is manipulated so that daily training activities are conducted with a success rate of approximately 80 percent. Training material is selected to meet the interests and vocabulary needs of the client. Listening activities are accompanied by information on strategies to manage communication situations. Appendixes 4–1 and 4–2 suggest materials for audiovisual training.

AUDITORY TRAINING

Most of the discussion of audiovisual training is applicable to auditory training. There are several reasons to include auditory-only activities in the audiologic rehabilitation process. New users of hearing aids must learn to decode a new signal. Emphasis on the amplified version of the speech signal without visual cues can demonstrate the benefit of hearing-aid use and speed the adjustment process. The visual cues of speech are not always available. Telephone use and darkness require auditory skills. People with visual impairments must develop auditory skills.

Typical auditory training activities are based on the following four levels of training suggested by Carhart (1960): (1) development of sound awareness; (2) development of gross sound discrimination; (3) development of broad speech discrimination; and (4) development of fine speech discrimination. Erber (1982) described a training program in terms of the linguistic unit (from syllables to paragraphs) and a hierarchy of responses to them (identification to comprehension). The typical older person with an acquired hearing loss does not require sound awareness training, but a few may require training to differentiate between speech and environmental sounds. Analytic activities are sometimes appropriate for speech discrimination. Same-different syllable drills or other analytic activities should be used only for phonemes that are problematic for the client. Confusion matrices, which plot clients' responses to phonemic stimuli (see Appendixes 2–4 and 2–5), can be useful to determine which phonemes require analytic work. The Garstecki (1981) training approach is useful in structuring auditory training activities. Appendixes 4–1 and 4–2 suggest auditory training materials and activities.

Auditory speech recognition in noise continues to be a problem for older listeners. Therefore, information concerning strategies for improving S/N should be included in the auditory training program. Listening training also can be productive. An older adult without a hearing loss may be able to function adequately with poor listening skills, but one with a hearing loss rarely can. The presence of the loss requires that full attention be paid to communication. An effective means of introducing the subject of listening and how it can affect speech recognition ability is to give the client a listening test. Such a test is provided in Table 4–1.

The author suggests that all statements are false.

TABLE 4–1 Listening Quiz

T ____ F ____	1.	Listening is largely a matter of intelligence.
T ____ F ____	2.	Speaking is a more important part of the communication process than listening.
T ____ F ____	3.	Listening requires little energy; it is easy.
T ____ F ____	4.	Listening is an automatic, involuntary reflex.
T ____ F ____	5.	Speakers can command listening within an audience.
T ____ F ____	6.	Hearing ability determines listening ability.
T ____ F ____	7.	The speaker is totally responsible for the success of communication.
T ____ F ____	8.	People listen every day. This daily practice eliminates the need for listening training.
T ____ F ____	9.	Competence in listening develops naturally.
T ____ F ____	10.	When you learned to read, you simultaneously learned to listen.
T ____ F ____	11.	Listening is only a matter of understanding the words of the speaker.

(Reprinted with permission from Barker 1971)

The telephone presents a special challenge to adults with hearing impairments (Erber, 1985; Castle, 1988). Practice of auditory training activities over the telephone during therapy sessions is often necessary.

EDUCATING SIGNIFICANT OTHERS

"Everyone mumbles."

"She always speaks to me from the other room, and she knows I can't hear."

"If I tell people I'm hard of hearing, they start shouting."

"We hardly talk anymore because it's so much trouble."

"I hate it when people say 'never mind' when I ask them to repeat."

"We never seem to go out anymore because she can't hear anything and feels left out."

"She always talks with that cigarette in her mouth."

"He always turns his back and walks away before he finishes what he's saying."

"I get so tired of repeating what everyone says all the time."

"My friends don't like to talk to me anymore—it's too much work."

Many adults with hearing impairments and their family members have the same complaints about one another. Family members, friends, co-workers, and caregivers of people with hearing impairments often have little understanding of hearing loss and even less knowledge of what they can do to make communication easier.

Hearing loss has a profound effect on communication and quality of life for clients and also for their frequent communication partners (Glass, 1991). Amplification may improve the situation, but problems remain, at least in difficult listening situations. Among the older population, it is common to learn that the client has never discussed the hearing loss or its effect with friends or family members.

It is therefore highly desirable to include family members and significant others in the rehabilitation process. Efforts in this regard, coupled with training the client, can have a dramatic effect on communication fluency and can reduce the frustration and irritation that occur when communication breaks down.

Significant others often have little understanding of the nature of hearing loss, the limitations of amplification and speechreading, or the effects of noise, distance, and reverberation on speech recognition. Increasing knowledge can help the significant others develop empathy for the partner with the hearing impairment, set realistic expectations for hearing aids in difficult listening situations, and make changes in the environment or in behavior that may reduce breakdowns. Information about the interactive nature of communication and mutual responsibility for success can motivate communication partners to learn specific skills that can minimize communication problems.

Tye-Murray and Schum (1994) suggest that the role of the clinician in providing conversational training to family members and to significant others is to foster empathy, appropriate speaking behaviors, message tailoring, and the use of verbal repair strategies. They state that this training is only one component of audiologic rehabilitation and that it is usually coordinated with services provided to the client.

Family participation in groups is helpful in increasing awareness because family members learn from the experiences and reactions of their peers as well as from the instructor. Clients and their partners can share problems and solutions while the clinician serves as facilitator. It is reassuring for many spouses to learn that other couples have many of the same experiences.

Table 4–2 provides an overview of topics appropriate to include in the education of family members and significant others. Not all items are appropriate for all people. Technical terminology should be avoided in this training. Appendixes 4–1 and 4–2 suggest resources for the education of significant others.

TABLE 4–2 Factors That Influence Speech Comprehension

ENVIRONMENTAL VARIABLES
Acoustics (distance, background noise, reverberation)

Lighting

Distractions

SPEAKER VARIABLES
Mouth movement

Rate of speech

Pitch and volume of voice

Familiarity

Accent

Objects in mouth

Expressiveness

Facial hair

PERSONAL VARIABLES
Hearing loss (audiogram, pure-tone thresholds, speech acoustics)

Speech recognition scores (in quiet, in noise)

Visual acuity

Alertness, fatigue

Concentration

Listening skills

Health

Erber's (1993) *Communication and Adult Hearing Loss* provides an excellent resource. This easy-to-read book can be lent to clients' significant others or used as a basis for presentations to them. It describes the interactive nature of communication, the ways hearing loss can interfere, and how specific behaviors can be changed to improve communication. *Speechreading: A Way to Improve Understanding* by Kaplan et al (1985) is also a valuable and practical resource.

Lists of guidelines or rules for people to use when speaking to a listener who is hard-of-hearing have been in use for many years. Trychin and Boone (1987) provide one such list. Applying specific suggestions can help family members with normal hearing reduce the number of communication breakdowns and to make their own repair efforts quick and efficient.

Caregivers of people with hearing impairments need special training, whether they are family members or staff of residential facilities. Improved awareness of how communication behaviors and environmental factors influence the success of communication can make the caretaker's job an easier one.

A clinician may occasionally find that problems or conflicts revealed during therapy are beyond his or her expertise. It is then necessary to refer a client or a couple for psychological counseling. If a psychologist or psychiatrist is not available who has an understanding of the mental health implications of acquired hearing loss, the clinician must educate the mental health professional as a significant other to that client. Trychin (1991) provided an excellent source of information about the mental health implications of hearing loss for professionals. In Chapter 5 of this book, Trychin discusses the counseling aspects of hearing care for the elderly. Trychin and Busacco (1991) provided a summary, written for a professional audience, of audiologic procedures, hearing technology, and environmental variables that affect speech recognition. These manuals can be helpful in planning in-service training or to lend to interested professionals.

People with hearing impairments can be their own advocates. They can assertively inform others of their communication needs, reinforce the good behaviors of others, and exhibit patience, because even well-informed and well-intentioned people forget at times. Because of the small amount of time that the significant other spends with the clinician, the client's efforts are essential for making long-term changes.

CONVERSATIONAL FLUENCY TRAINING

Erber (1985; 1988; 1993) added the concept of conversational training to auditory training with a stated goal of developing the client's metalinguistic skills. Erber described a successful conversational exchange as one in which all who participate share a common language, are cooperative and want to communicate, and are willing to follow the complex set of socially acceptable procedures for human communication. To the degree that hearing impairment or poor listening habits interfere with the spontaneity of the interchange, conversational fluency is decreased. The satisfaction that participants receive from a conversation is related to the fluency of that conversation.

In conversational fluency training, video tapes of conversations can be reviewed to examine communication behaviors such as turn taking, maintaining the topic, use of clarification procedures, and pragmatic conventions. Contingencies in conversations can be described; comments or questions by one's communication partner can influence the content and the form of the response (what is said and how it is said). Clients can be given the opportunity to practice asking specific, response-limiting questions in a simulated conversation using QUEST?AR (Erber 1985).

QUEST?AR is a conversational training technique in which the instructor specifies a topic of conversation, and the client asks 30 related questions (Table 4–3). Each topic is a place presumably visited recently by the clinician. The sequence of questions allows the client to find out about the trip. The place is clearly specified to the client (by audiovisual presentation or in writing). The client then asks each question in sequence, obtaining an answer before proceeding. The client should request repetition or repair strategies if he or she does not understand the instructor's answer. When both participants treat the activity as if it were a real conversation, strategies can be applied naturally. Other clients or family members can act as the respondent for practice in modifying their answers after requests for clarification. The QUEST?AR package includes a booklet that contains the written questions on separate pages. A printed list of the questions works just as well in providing almost natural practice in interactive conversational skills.

TABLE 4–3 QUEST?AR (QUESTions for Aural Rehabilitation)

TOPIC

Where did you go? (eg, grocery store, vacation cruise, party, museum)

QUESTIONS

1. Why did you go there?
2. When did you go?
3. How many people went with you?
4. Who were they?
5. What did you take with you?
6. Where is the [place you went]?
7. How did you get there?
8. What did you see on the way?
9. What time did you get there?
10. What did you do first?
11. What did you see?
12. How many? What color?
13. What happened at the [place where you went]?

TABLE 4–3 QUEST?AR (QUESTions for Aural Rehabilitation) (continued)

14.	What else did you do?
15.	What were other people doing at the [place where you went]?
16.	What was the most interesting thing that you saw?
17.	What was the most interesting thing that you did?
18.	What did you buy?
19.	What kind? What flavor? What color?
20.	How much did it cost?
21.	Did anything unusual happen? What?
22.	How long did you stay?
23.	What did you do just before you came home?
24.	When did you leave?
25.	How did you get home?
26.	What happened on the way home?
27.	What time did you get home?
28.	How did you feel then?
29.	When are you going back?
30.	Do you think that I should go there sometime? Why?

(Reprinted from Erber 1985)

TOPICON (Erber, 1988) is another procedure for simulating conversation in the therapy environment. It is a conversational sampling, evaluation, and practice procedure and is described in Chapter 2. TOPICON is appropriate for use when the structure provided by the specific questions in QUEST?AR is no longer needed. The clinician may intentionally violate rules of good communication to degrade the signal and force the client to use strategies. After each session, remedial strategies chosen (or overlooked) by the client can be noted and their appropriateness and effectiveness can be discussed. The assessment and the discussion between the client and clinician that follows the use of TOPICON can provide information about the direction of subsequent therapy activities.

Background noise of different types and intensities should be added as the client's conversational fluency in quiet increases. Compact disks (Appendixes 4–1 and 4–2) offer a wide variety of background noises to approximate the noises that a client finds problematic. Visual distractions can be introduced to make conversational practice more realistic. Appendixes 4–1 and 4–2 suggest materials related to conversational fluency training.

STRATEGIES TRAINING

Clients with hearing losses and those who communicate with them use a variety of strategies to reduce communication breakdowns or repair them when they inevitably occur. These strategies give the person with the hearing impairment a sense of control in difficult listening situations. The strategies provide concrete behaviors that can be applied as the client assumes responsibility for improving communication. Kaplan et al (1985) provided a concise description of strategies and the assertiveness needed to use them. Anticipatory strategies can be used before an event to minimize the number of breakdowns that occur. However, no amount of planning completely prevents communication breakdowns for older adults with hearing impairments. Therefore, repair strategies are needed. Castle (1988) provided a summary of strategies as they apply to telephone use. Appendixes 4–1 and 4–2 present materials related to strategies training, and Table 4–4 summarizes anticipatory and repair strategies.

TABLE 4–4 Strategies for Use by People with Hearing Impairments

ANTICIPATORY STRATEGIES

Anticipate possible vocabulary

Anticipate possible dialogue and its sequence

Anticipate environmental problems

Anticipate questions that may be asked

Decide what information is needed

Consider how to be assertive

Plan questions to ask

Decide how to narrow and specify questions

Plan how to modify the environment

Consider how to be assertive

REPAIR STRATEGIES

Repeat

Summarize

Rephrase

Say key words

Spell key word

Gesture

Ask a specific question

Ask a general question

Write a brief message (focus on key words)

Say each digit individually (for numbers)

TABLE 4–4 Strategies for Use by People with Hearing Impairments (continued)

TELEPHONE STRATEGIES

Ask for confirmation of understanding

Repeat what was heard

Use code words (A as in alpha, B as in beta)

Ask speaker to say alphabet and stop at correct letter

Ask for numbers to be spoken individually or spelled

Ask talker to count from zero to the correct number and stop

(Anticipatory and repair strategies adapted from Kaplan et al 1985; telephone strategies adapted from Castle 1988)

Tye-Murray et al (1992) surveyed members of Self Help for Hard of Hearing People (SHHH) and found that the strategy most commonly used was repetition. Gagne and Wyllie (1989), however, found that the simple repetition strategy was less successful than more specific strategies. Gagné et al (1990) also found that requests for simple repetitions were the least well received by communication partners with normal hearing. Listeners with hearing losses who made specific requests (such as repeating the portion they understood and guessing) were rated higher than those who made more general requests (such as "huh?" and "say again."). This finding suggests that clinicians should emphasize training their clients to use strategies that provide information to or make specific requests of the speaker.

Several activities can be used to train clients and to evaluate the strategies they use. Speech-tracking (De Filippo & Scott, 1978), described earlier, requires the speechreader to make requests of the speaker. Erber's conversational fluency training procedures, such as QUEST?AR (Erber, 1985) and TOPICON (Erber, 1988) can also be useful in providing opportunities to practice the use of strategies.

Tye-Murray et al (1988) developed an interactive video disk program that uses computer-assisted instruction to provide clients with practice in choosing and requesting strategies. The use of this type of system should increase as the required hardware becomes available.

CREATING A POSITIVE COMMUNICATION ENVIRONMENT

Most older adults with hearing impairments can specify situations they find to cause problems. Just as they are often unable to apply strategies, older people are also frequently unable to manipulate the environment to improve communication. Family members and significant others are even more unlikely to understand that the factors listed in Table 4–3 can have a strong impact on the ability of a person with a hearing impairment to understand speech. Educating significant others plays an important role in creating a positive communication environment.

When clients and their communication partners understand the variables, they are better able to make changes in situations in which modifications are possible and to develop realistic expectations and apply compensatory strategies in situations in which communication is difficult. Activities can be created to encourage people with hearing impairments to use this information to make changes in their environment, to make informed decisions about public places to patronize or avoid, and to make choices about the best possible time or place to position themselves in unfavorable environments.

Assertiveness Training

Rationale

I have found through clinical experience that many older adults with hearing impairments believe the responsibility for communication is entirely their own and that they should not ask others to modify their behaviors to accommodate for the hearing loss. Many others are not reluctant to inform others of their hearing loss and give suggestions, but they do not necessarily do so in a manner that inspires cooperation from the partner. Assertiveness training can be of benefit when it improves clients' willingness and ability to admit to a hearing problem, explain the problem to others when appropriate, and suggest ways to improve communication (Abrahamson, 1991).

Kaplan et al (1985) stated that passive communication behaviors can result in frustration, isolation, feelings of inadequacy, and reduced self-esteem. Rocky Stone, writing as the Executive Director of SHHH, stated that "Many problems, worries and anguish stemming from hearing impairment can be avoided by the cultivation of an honest and open method of communication, with insistence on the right to understand and be understood" (DiMichael, 1985, p. 3). Assertiveness training can effectively foster this open method of communication, but care should be taken in introducing this topic to older adults. They may not be as comfortable as are younger adults with stating their needs and making demands on others. Discussions are not sufficient. Clients need an opportunity to practice new skills in a safe, structured environment if they are to change a lifelong history of passive communication behaviors.

Role-playing

Role-playing in a group can provide practice of new assertiveness skills. Trychin and Bonvillian (1992) provided a workbook with scripts and instructions that allow nonprofessional actors to create and present skits that depict situations that involve communication and hearing loss. Skits can provide a nonthreatening means of introducing topics that can be emotionally charged. Watching people act out a problem situation is often more informative than a discussion. Acting out problem situations gives the actors practice in using repair strategies in an assertive manner. Observers can provide feedback on the choice and effectiveness of the strategy and how the interaction was perceived.

Assertiveness exists on a continuum with aggressiveness. Schum (1993) observed that people with hearing impairments are sometimes perceived as being angry because of an inability to modulate their assertiveness. Clients are told in therapy to be assertive and attempt to do so, but their efforts (eg, verbal and nonverbal behavior, tone of voice) are sometimes interpreted as anger. Peers can provide feedback on how the client appears in the role-playing activities. Role-plays by a group over a period of several weeks can be an effective means of developing assertiveness skills that will foster cooperation from communication partners. As these skills emerge and the clients' confidence in using them grows, the clinician can make homework assignments for clients to use assertiveness in specified situations outside the class. The outcomes of these assignments are then discussed in class.

Consumer Organizations

Several consumer organizations provide valuable resources for older adults with hearing impairments and their families. Educational materials are available at minimal cost on a wide variety of topics ranging from hearing aids, assistive devices, social and psychologic effects of hearing loss, causes, treatment, and adjustment to tinnitus and speechreading. Several of these organizations are listed in Appendix 4–3. Additional sources of public education materials are also included.

Lieberth (1992) described the success of volunteers from a local SHHH group in providing service to adults with hearing impairments. Volunteers were trained to share information about hearing loss and strategies for coping with hearing loss. With the audiologist acting as case manager, volunteers saw clients in groups in the clinic or in the clients' homes. This program was well received, and Lieberth is collecting longitudinal data on its success.

Besides providing education, consumer organizations can provide motivation for older adults with hearing impairments to become advocates. Taking an active role in the political issues related to hearing loss can help people with hearing impairments increase their sense of control. Active older people with hearing losses can play an important role in educating the general public about the effects of hearing loss, and they can have a strong influence on the implementation of the Americans with Disabilities Act of 1990 (Abrahamson, 1991).

Consumer organizations provide clients with emotional support and peer interaction. Family members may receive similar support and enjoy contact with other couples or people with hearing losses. Group members provide role models of adults who manage their hearing losses effectively, maintain close personal relations, and lead productive lives.

ASSESSING THE EFFECTIVENESS OF AUDIOLOGIC REHABILITATION PROGRAMS

The roots of audiology as a profession are in the auditory rehabilitation needs of veterans with hearing impairments as they returned from World War II. Over time, increasingly sophisticated equipment and procedures for diagnosis and research became the focus of the profession. The difficulty of quantifying a client's successful personal management of hearing loss and documenting measurable improvement as the result of participation in audiologic rehabilitation programs has been a contributing factor in a trend away from rehabilitation. Aside from anecdotal reports, documentation of benefit from audiologic rehabilitation (except hearing-aid fitting) has been elusive. Many audiologists do not provide these necessary services because objective measurements of audiologic rehabilitation are more difficult to quantify than a 20-dB shift in threshold at 1000 Hz. Audiologists who do offer these services often feel unable to quantify or otherwise document the improvement that their clients and their clinical experience tells them exists. Chapter 2 provides a comprehensive review of evaluation of audiologic rehabilitation.

The development of cochlear implants has revived interest in audiologic rehabilitation. The United States Food and Drug Administration, in granting licenses for cochlear implants, requires that specific treatment protocols be followed. Longitudinal studies of the performance of patients who have received implants must be completed. Analogous investigations of the success of rehabilitation programs for people with less severe hearing losses are needed. Evaluation protocols, developed for use with implant candidates and recipients, can be modified for use with clients with less severe losses.

CONCLUSION

For a large number of adults, hearing care services must continue past the point of hearing-aid fitting. Montgomery (1991) stated that participation in a group is the most effective way to ensure that hearing aids will be worn after they are purchased. For some clients, additional perceptual training is needed. In many cases, common-sense solutions to communication problems do not present themselves to people with hearing losses or their frequent communication partners. For many, training in ways to improve communication may be as important as the choice of appropriate amplification in improving quality of life.

Ross (1992) stated that

> Professionals engaged in the practice of A/R are still searching for professional respectability, attempting simultaneously to develop supportable procedures and material, to convince their colleagues and clients of the need and potential efficacy of A/R and to lobby for service-delivery models by which A/R could be funded by third-party payers (p. 2).

It is hoped that the information presented in this chapter will encourage clinicians to offer rehabilitation services as part of comprehensive hearing care and provide practical considerations for doing so.

REFERENCES

Abrahamson, J.E. (1991). Teaching coping strategies: A client education approach to aural rehabilitation. *Journal of the Academy of Rehabilitative Audiology, 24,* 43-53.

Alpiner, J.G. (1982). *Handbook of adult rehabilitative audiology* (2nd ed.) Baltimore: Williams & Wilkins.

American Speech-Language-Hearing Association (1993). Preferred practice patterns for the professions of speech-language pathology and audiology. *ASHA, 35,* (Suppl. 11).

AUDITEC of St. Louis. (1981). *Auditory training lessons.* St. Louis: AUDITEC of St. Louis.

Barker, L.L. (1971). *Listening behavior.* Englewood Cliffs: Prentice-Hall.

Binnie, C.A., Montgomery, A.A., & Jackson, P.L. (1974). Auditory and visual contributions to the perception of consonants. *Journal of Speech and Hearing Research, 17,* 619-630.

Carhart, R. (1960). Auditory training. In. H. Davis & R. Silverman (Eds.), *Hearing and deafness* (2nd ed.) (pp. 368-386). New York: Holt, Rinehart & Winston.

Castle, D.L. (1988). *Telephone strategies: A technical and practical guide for hard of hearing people.* Bethesda: SHHH Press.

Cherry, R., & Rubinstein, A. (1988) Speechreading instruction for adults: Issues and practices. *Volta Review, 90,* 289-306.

Compton, C. (1991). *Assistive devices: Doorways to independence* [videotape]. Washington: Gallaudet University.

De Filippo, C.L. (1988). Tracking for speechreading training. In C.L. De Filippo & D.G. Sims (Eds.), *New reflections on speechreading.* Washington: Alexander Graham Bell Association for the Deaf.

De Filippo, C.L., & Scott, B.L. (1978). A method for training and evaluating the reception of ongoing speech. *Journal of the Acoustical Society of America, 63,* 1186-1192.

DiMichael, S.G. (1985). *Assertiveness training for persons who are hard of hearing.* Bethesda: SHHH Press.

Erber, N.P. (1982). *Auditory training.* Washington: Alexander Graham Bell Association for the Deaf.

Erber, N.P. (1985). *Telephone communication and hearing impairment.* San Diego: College-Hill Press.

Erber, N.P. (1988). *Communication therapy for hearing-impaired adults.* Abbotsford: Clavis.

Erber, N.P. (1993). *Communication and adult hearing loss.* Abbotsford: Clavis.

Feeham, P.J., Samuelson, R.A., & Seymour, D.T. (1982). *Clues: Speechreading for Adults.* Tigard: C.C. Publications.

Gagné, J.P., Stelmacovich, P., & Yovetich, W.S. (1990). Reactions to requests for clarification used by hearing-impaired individuals. Presented at the Academy of Rehabilitative Audiology Summer Institute, June 8-10, 1990, Howey-in-the-Hills, Fla.

Gagné, J.P., & Wyllie, K.A. (1989). Relative effectiveness of three repair strategies on the visual-identification of misperceived words. *Ear and Hearing, 10,* 368-374.

Garstecki, D.C. (1981). Auditory-visual training paradigm for hearing impaired adults. *Journal of the Academy of Rehabilitative Audiology, 14,* 223-238.

Glass, L. E. (1991). Psychosocial aspects of hearing loss in adulthood. In H. Orlean (Ed.), *Adjustment to adult hearing loss.* San Diego: Singular.

Greenwald, A.B. (1984). *Lipreading made easy* [videotape]. Washington: Alexander Graham Bell Association for the Deaf.

Hardick, E. (1977). Aural rehabilitation programs for the aged can be successful. *Journal of the Academy of Rehabilitative Audiology, 10,* 51-67.

Jeffers, J., & Barley, M. (1976). *Speechreading (lipreading).* Springfield: Thomas.

Johnson, D.D., & Caccamise, F. (1982) Visual assessment of hearing-impaired persons: Options and implications for the future. *Journal of the Academy of Rehabilitative Audiology, 15,* 22-40.

Kaplan, H.F., Bally, S., & Garretson, C. (1985). *Speechreading: A way to improve understanding* (2nd ed.). Washington: Gallaudet University Press.

Kelly, L. (1993). The readability of hearing aid brochures. Presented at the Academy of Rehabilitative Audiology Summer Institute, June 10-13, Howey-in-the-Hills, Fla.

Lesner, S.A., & Kricos, P.B. (1991). Audiologic rehabilitation: Candidacy, assessment, and management. In D. Ripich (Ed.), *Geriatric communication disorders* (pp. 439-461). Austin: Pro-Ed.

Lesner, S.A. (1992). Hearing disorder management in patients with presbycusis. *Hearing Instruments, 45,* 11-12.

Lieberth, A.K. (1992). New directions in adult aural rehabilitation. *Tejas, 18,* 37-39.

Luterman, D.M. (1991). *Counseling the communicatively disordered and their families* (2nd ed.) Austin: Pro-Ed.

Montgomery, A.A. (1984). Streamlining the aural rehabilitation process. *Hearing Instruments, 35,* 46-49.

Montgomery, A.A. (1991). Aural rehabilitation: Review and preview. In G.A. Studebaker, F.H. Bess & L.B. Beck (Eds.), *The Vanderbilt hearing-aid report. II.* Parkton: York.

Ordman, K.A., & Ralli, M.P. (1976). *What people say.* Washington: Alexander Graham Bell Association for the Deaf.

Owens, E., & Raggio, M. (1987). The UCSF tracking procedure for evaluation and training of speech reception by hearing-impaired adults. *Journal of Speech and Hearing Disorders, 52,* 120-128.

Owens, E., & Telleen, C. (1981). Tracking as an aural rehabilitative process. *Journal of the Academy of Rehabilitative Audiology, 14,* 259-273.

Pelson, R.O., & Prather, W.F. (1974). Effects of visual message-related cues, age and hearing impairment on speechreading performance. *Journal of Speech and Hearing Research, 17,* 518-525.

Perry, A.L. (1977). A lipreading curriculum for adults. *Volta Review, 7,* 381-393.

Roberts, S.D., & Bryant, J.D. (1992). Establishing counseling goals in rehabilitative audiology. *Journal of the Academy of Rehabilitative Audiology, 25,* 81-97.

Ross, M. (1992). *Aural rehabilitation: Materials, procedures, and implications.* Durham: National Institute of Disability and Rehabilitation Research, University of New Hampshire.

Schum, R. (1993). Psychological perspective on hearing impairment: Needs and intervention. Presented at the Academy of Rehabilitative Audiology Summer Institute, June 10-13, 1993, Howey-in-the-Hills, Fla.

Trychin, S. (1987). *Communication rules for hard of hearing people* [videotape]. Bethesda: SHHH Press.

Trychin, S. (1991). *Manual for mental health professionals. II. Basic information for providing services to hard of hearing people and their families.* Washington: Gallaudet University Press.

Trychin, S., & Bonvillian, B. (1992). *Actions speak louder: Tips for putting on skits related to hearing loss.* Bethesda: SHHH Press.

Trychin, S., & Boone, M. (1987). *Communication rules for hard of hearing people.* Bethesda: SHHH Press.

Trychin, S., & Busacco, S. (1991). *Manual for mental health professionals. I. Psychosocial challenges faced by hard of hearing people.* Washington: Gallaudet University Press.

Tye-Murray, N., Purdy, S., and Woodworth, G. (1992). Reported use of communication strategies by SHHH members: Client, talker, and situational variables. *Journal of Speech and Hearing Research, 35,* 708-717.

Tye-Murray, N., & Schum L. (1994). Conversation training for frequent communication partners. *Journal of the Academy of Rehabilitative Audiology Monograph, 27,* 209-223.

Tye-Murray, N., Tyler, R. S., Bong, R., & Nares, T. (1988). Computerized laser videodisk programs for training speechreading and assertive communication behaviors. *Journal of the Academy of Rehabilitative Audiology, 21,* 143-152.

United States National Health Survey (1968). *Monocular-binocular visual acuity of adults.* Public Health Service Publication No. 100, Series 11, No. 30, 1960-1962. Washington: United States Government Printing Office.

Wayner, D.S. (1990a). *The hearing aid handbook: Clinician's guide to client orientation.* Washington: Gallaudet University Press.

Wayner, D.S. (1990b). *The hearing aid handbook: User's guide for adults.* Washington: Gallaudet University Press.

Appendix 4–1

Materials for Use in Audiologic Rehabilitation of Older Adults

TRAINING CATEGORY	Auditory	Speechreading	Audiovisual	Strategies	Conversational Fluency	Assertiveness	Patient Education	Significant Other	Care-giver	Professional In-service	Hearing Aid or Assistive Listening Device Use	Lending Library
BOOKS												
Armbruster & Gaydos (1981)											X	X
Berger (1972)		X										
Broberg (1963)		X										
Broberg (1984)		X										
Brinson (1986)							X	X	X		X	X
Bruhn (1949)		X										
Bunger (1961)		X										
Castle (1984)	X							X				X
Castle (1988)	X		X					X				X
Erickson (1989)		X										
Feeham et al (1982)		X										
Fisher (1978)		X										
Flexer et al (1990)			X	X	X					X	X	X*
Gallaudet University & ASHA (1988)								X	X	X		
Greenwald (1984)		X										X
Hallman (1989)							X					X

TRAINING CATEGORY	Auditory	Speechreading	Audiovisual	Strategies	Conversational Fluency	Assertiveness	Patient Education	Significant Other	Care-giver	Professional In-service	Hearing Aid or Assistive Listening Device Use	Lending Library
BOOKS												
Haug & Haug (1977)	X	X	X	X			X					X
Hazard (1971)		X										
Himber (1989)			X				X	X			X	X
Jacobs (1981)		X	X				X					X
Jeffers & Barley (1971)		X										
Jeffers & Barley (1979)		X										
Kaplan et al (1985)		X	X	X		X	X					X
Kisor (1990)												X*
Light (1978)	X											
Luey & Per-Lee (1983)				X			X					X
Marcus (1985)		X										X
Ordman & Ralli (1976)		X										
Orlans (1985)				X				X		X		X*
Rezen & Hausman (1985)				X		X	X	X	X			X
Sayre (1980a)	X	X	X	X			X	X				X
Sayre (1980b)							X	X	X			X
Scott (1979)	X											X
Shimon (1982)							X	X		X		
Smith & Karp (1978)	X								X			X
Trychin (1986a)							X	X				X
Trychin (1986b)							X			X		
Trychin (1987a)				X		X	X	X	X	X		X
Trychin (1987b)				X		X	X	X				X
Trychin (1988)				X		X	X	X	X	X		X
Trychin (1991)				X		X	X*			X		X*
Trychin & Boone (1987)				X		X	X	X	X	X		X
Trychin & Busacco (1991)				X		X	X	X	X	X		X*
Trychin & Wright (1989)							X	X				X
Whitehurst (1964)	X	X	X									
Whitehurst (1986)	X											

TRAINING CATEGORY	Auditory	Speechreading	Audiovisual	Strategies	Conversational Fluency	Assertiveness	Patient Education	Significant Other	Care-giver	Professional In-service	Hearing Aid or Assistive Listening Device Use	Lending Library
VIDEO TAPES												
Assistive Devices: Doorways to Independence							X	X	X	X	X	X
Assistive Devices for Hearing-Impaired Persons							X	X	X	X	X	X
Beyond Hearing Loss: Resource Guide for Senior Citizens							X	X	X		X	X
Communication Rules for Hard of Hearing People				X		X	X	X	X			X
Did I Do That?				X		X	X	X				X
I Only Hear You When I See Your Face							X	X	X			X
Learning Speechreading		X										X
Lipreading Made Easy		X										X
Read My Lips		X										X
Relaxation Training for Hard of Hearing People							X					X
Speechreading Counseling		X					X			X		X
Speechreading: Survival on the Job & Social Situation Sentences		X										X
AUDIO TAPES												
Auditory Training Lessons	X											X
Getting Through: A Guide to Better Understanding								X	X	X		X
Relaxation Training for People Who Are Hard of Hearing							X					X
Sound Hearing								X	X	X		X
Telecoil Evaluation Procedure	X											
PERIODICALS												
SHHH							X	X				X
Tinnitus Today							X	X				X
Hearing Health							X	X				X

TRAINING CATEGORY	Auditory	Speechreading	Audiovisual	Strategies	Conversational Fluency	Assertiveness	Patient Education	Significant Other	Care-giver	Professional In-service	Hearing Aid or Assistive Listening Device Use	Lending Library
COMPUTER PROGRAMS												
Cox et al (1987)	X		X									
Kopra et al (1984)		X	X									
Palmer & Garstecki (1988)											X	
Pichora-Fuller & Bengurel (1990)		x										
COMPACT DISKS												
Sound Effects (1992)	X		X									
OTHER MATERIALS												
Read My Lips (game)								X				X
QUEST?AR Communication Kit	X	X	X	X	X							

*Clinician judgment must be used in selecting materials for home use by patients and family members, based on reading level, technical content, and individual interests.

Appendix 4–2

Materials for Use in Audiologic Rehabilitation of Older Adults

Books

Armbruster, J.M., & Gaydos, J. (1981). *How to get the most out of your hearing aid.* Washington: Alexander Graham Bell Association for the Deaf.

Berger, K.W. (1972). *Speechreading principles and methods.* Kent: Herald.

Brinson, W. (1986). *Deafness in the adult: What hearing loss means and what can be done about it.* Wellingborough: Thorsons.

Broberg, R.F. (1963). *Stories and games for easy lipreading practice* (2nd ed.) Washington: Alexander Graham Bell Association for the Deaf.

Broberg, R.F. (1984). *The lipreaders' calendar: Practice material to take you round the year in 40 days.* Washington: Alexander Graham Bell Association for the Deaf.

Bruhn, M.E. (1949) *The Mueller-Walle method of lipreading for the hard of hearing.* Washington: Volta Bureau.

Bunger, A.M. (1961). *Speech reading Jena method: A textbook with lesson plans in full development for hard of hearing adults and discussion of adaptations for hard of hearing and deaf children.* Danvillle: Interstate.

Castle, D.L. (1984). *Telephone training for hearing-impaired persons: Amplified telephones, TDDs, codes.* Washington: Alexander Graham Bell Association for the Deaf.

Castle, D.L. (1988). *Telephone strategies: A technical and practical guide for hard-of-hearing people.* Bethesda: SHHH Publications.

Erickson, J.G. (1989). *Speechreading: A guide to understanding.* Washington: Alexander Graham Bell Association for the Deaf.

Feeham, P.J., Samuelsen, R.A., & Seymour, D.T. (1982). *Clues: Speech reading for adults.* Tigard: C.C. Publications.

Fisher, M. (1978). *Lively lipreading lessons.* Washington: Alexander Graham Bell Association for the Deaf.

Flexer, C., Wray, D., & Leavit, R. (1990). *How the student with hearing loss can succeed in college: A handbook for students, families and professionals.* Washington: Alexander Graham Bell Association for the Deaf.

Gallaudet University & American Speech-Language-Hearing Association (1988). *When hearing fades: Community health center response to hearing loss in elderly clients: a training guide.*

Greenwald, A.B. (1984). *Lipreading made easy.* Washington: Alexander Graham Bell Association for the Deaf.

Hallman, R. (1989). *Living with tinnitus.* Washington: Alexander Graham Bell Association for the Deaf.

Haug, O., & Haug, S. (1977). *Help for the hard-of-hearing: A speech reading and auditory training manual for home and professionally guided training.* Springfield: Thomas.

Hazard, E. (1971). *Lipreading for the oral deaf and hard-of hearing person.* Springfield: Thomas.

Himber, C. (1989). *How to survive hearing loss.* Washington: Gallaudet University Press.

Jacobs, M. (1981). *Associational cues.* Rochester: Rochester Institute of Technology.

Jeffers, J., & Barley, M. (1971). *Speechreading (lipreading).* Springfield: Thomas.

Jeffers, J., & Barley, M. (1979). *Look, now hear this.* Springfield: Thomas.

Kaplan, H., Bally, S., & Garretson, C. (1985). *Speechreading: A way to improve understanding* (2nd ed.) Washington: Gallaudet University Press.

Kisor, H. (1990). *What's that pig outdoors?: A memoir of deafness.* New York: Hill & Wang.

Light, J.B. (1978). *The joy of listening: An auditory training program.* Washington: Alexander Graham Bell Association for the Deaf.

Luey, H.S., & Per-Lee, M.S. (1983). *What should I do now? Problems and adaptations of the deafened adult.* Washington: National Academy of Gallaudet College.

Marcus, I.S. (1985). *Your eyes hear for you: A self-help course in speechreading.* Bethesda: SHHH Publications.

Ordman, K.A., & Ralli, M.P. (1976). *What people say.* Washington: Alexander Graham Bell Association for the Deaf.

Orlans, H. (Ed.) (1985). *Adjustment to adult hearing loss.* Baltimore: College Hill Press.

Rezen, S.V., & Hausman, C. (1985). *Coping with hearing loss: A guide for adults & their families.* New York: Dembner.

Sayre, J.M. (1980a). *Handbook for the hearing impaired older adult: An individualized program.* Danville: Interstate.

Sayre, J.M. (1980b). *Helping the older adult with an acquired hearing loss: Suggestions and techniques for clinicians, audiologists, and others working with the adult hearing-impaired.* Danville: Interstate.

Scott, D. (1979). *Learning to listen again: Home course for adults with hearing loss.* Toronto: Canadian Hearing Society.

Shimon, D.A. (1992). *Coping with hearing loss and hearing aids.* San Diego: Singular.

Smith, C.R., & Karp, A. (1978). *A workbook in auditory training for adults: With a special section on the institutionalized geriatric patient.* Springfield: Thomas.

Trychin, S. (1986a). *Relaxation training for hard of hearing people: Trainee's manual.* Bethesda: SHHH Publications.

Trychin, S. (1986b). *Relaxation training for hard of hearing people: Practitioner's manual.* Bethesda: SHHH Publications.

Trychin, S. (1987a). *Did I do that?: Manual.* Bethesda: SHHH Publications.

Trychin, S. (1987b). *Stress management.* SHHH Information Series No. 203. Bethesda: SHHH Publications.

Trychin, S. (1988). *So that's the problem.* Bethesda: SHHH Publications.

Trychin, S. (1991). *Manual for mental health professionals. II. Psycho-social challenges faced by hard of hearing people.* Washington: Gallaudet University Press.

Trychin, S., & Boone, M. (1987a). *Communication rules for hard of hearing people: Manual.* Bethesda: SHHH Publications.

Trychin, S., & Busacco, D. (1991). *Manual for mental health professionals. I. Basic information for providing services to hard of hearing people and their families.* Washington: Gallaudet University Press.

Trychin, S., & Wright, F. (1989). *Is THAT what you think?* Bethesda: SHHH Publications.

Tucker, B.P., & Goldstein, B.A. (1990). *Legal rights of persons with disabilities: An analysis of federal law.* Washington: Alexander Graham Bell Association for the Deaf.

Whitehurst, M.W. (1964). *Integrated lessons in lipreading and auditory training.* Armonk: Hearing Rehabilitation.

Whitehurst, M.W. (1986). *Listen to me: Auditory exercises for adults.* Washington: Alexander Graham Bell Association for the Deaf.

Video Tapes

Assistive devices: Doorways to independence (1991). Cynthia Compton, Gallaudet University, 800 Florida Ave, NE, Washington, DC 20002. Available through Academy of Dispensing Audiologists (800) 454-8629. Tape and manual.

Assistive devices for hearing-impaired persons (1987). New York League for the Hard of Hearing, 71 West 23rd St, New York, NY 10010-4162, 212-741-7650 (voice) or 212-255-1932 (TTY).

Beyond hearing loss: Resource guide for senior citizens (1991). Johns Hopkins Center for Hearing and Balance, 601 N. Caroline St., Baltimore, MD 21203, 410-955-3403.

Communication rules for hard of hearing people (1987). S. Trychin & M. Boone. SHHH Publications, 7910 Woodmont Ave., Suite 1200, Bethesda, MD 20814, 301-657-2248.

Did I do that? (1987). S. Trychin. SHHH Publications, 7910 Woodmont Ave., Suite 1200, Bethesda, MD 20814, 301-657-2248.

I only hear you when I see your face (1988). Produced by Hope for Hearing Foundation. Available from Alexander Graham Bell Association for the Deaf, 3417 Volta Pl, NW, Washington, DC 20007-2778, 202-337-5220.

Learning speechreading (1989). Speech and Hearing Technologies, 862 Kelsey Ct, Centerville, OH 45458, 513-435-1407. Series of four video tapes.

Lipreading made easy (1984). A.B. Greenwald. Alexander Graham Bell Association for the Deaf, 3417 Volta Pl, NW, Washington, DC 20007-2778, 202-337-5220.

Read my lips (1988). Speechreading Laboratory, Inc., PO Box 648130, Mustang, OK 73064. Series of six video tapes for home use, booklet, and score sheets.

Relaxation training for hard of hearing people (1986). S. Trychin. SHHH Publications, 7910 Woodmont Ave., Suite 1200, Bethesda, MD 20814, 301-657-2248.

Speechreading counseling (1989). Speech & Hearing Technologies, 862 Kelsey Court, Centerville, OH 45458, 513-435-1407. Series of four video-tapes.

Speechreading: Survival on the job and social situation sentences (1987). M. Jacobs. Alexander Graham Bell Association for the Deaf, 3417 Volta Pl, NW, Washington, DC 20007-2778, 202-337-5220. Eleven tapes plus workbooks.

Audio Tapes

Auditory training lessons (1982). AUDITEC of St. Louis, 2515 S. Big Bend Blvd., St. Louis, MO 63143, 800-669-9065.

Getting through: A guide to better understanding (1986). SHHH Publications, 7910 Woodmont Ave., Suite 1200, Bethesda, MD 20814, 301-657-2248.

Relaxation training for people who are hard of hearing (1986). SHHH Publications, 7910 Woodmont Ave., Suite 1200, Bethesda, MD 20814, 301-657-2248

Sound hearing: Or . . . hearing what you miss (1989). S.H. Collins. Garlic Press, 100 Hillview Ln., #2, Eugene, OR 97408, 503-345-0063.

Telecoil evaluation procedure: An audio tape hearing aid evaluation to determine the benefit of a hearing aid for telephone use (1987). M.J. Wallber & D.J. MacKenzie. AUDITEC of St. Louis, 2515 S. Big Bend Blvd., St. Louis, MO 63143, 800-669-9065.

Periodicals

Hearing health: The voice on hearing issues. Voice International Publications Inc., PO Box 2663, Corpus Christi, TX 78403-2663. Subscription $14.00 per year.

SHHH: The Journal of Self Help for Hard of Hearing People. SHHH Publications, 7910 Woodmont Ave., Suite 1200, Bethesda, MD 20814. Cost included in membership.

Tinnitus Today: The Journal of the American Tinnitus Association. PO Box 5, Portland, OR 97207. Cost included in membership.

Computer Programs

Cox, R M , Alexander, G.C., & Gilmore. C. (1987). *Connected speech test.* Memphis Speech and Hearing Center, 807 Jefferson Ave., Memphis, TN 38105, 901-678-5800.

Kopra, L.L., Kopra, M.A., Abrahamson, J.E., & Dunlop, R.J. (1984). *University of Texas drill and practice sentences for computer-assisted instruction in lipreading.* Department of Communication Sciences and Disorders, University of Texas at Austin, CMA 2.200, Austin, TX 78712, 512-471-3841. Video disk, software, and documentation.

Palmer, C.V., & Garstecki, D.C. (1988). A computer spreadsheet for locating assistive devices. *Journal of the Academy of Rehabilitative Audiology, 21,* 158-175.

Pichora-Fuller, M., & Benguerel, A. (1990). The design of CAST (computer aided speechreading training). *Journal of Speech & Hearing Research, 34,* 202-212.

Compact Disk

Sound Effects (1992). Micro Sound Products, 1955 W Texas, Suite 7-327, Fairfield, CA 94533, 707-428-6363. Four compact disks with more than 250 environmental sounds.

Other Materials

QUEST?AR Communication Kit (1988). Clavis Publishing, Abbotsford, Victoria, Australia. Available from Hear You Are, Inc., 4 Musconetcong Ave., Stanhope, NJ 07874, 201-347-7662.

Read My Lips: The Wild Party Game of Unspoken Words. New Brunswick, NJ: Pressman Toy Corp.

Appendix 4–3

Consumer Organizations

Alexander Graham Bell Association for the Deaf
3417 Volta Place, NW
Washington, DC 20007-2778
202-337-5220

American Tinnitus Association
PO Box 5
Portland, OR 97207
503-248-9985

Association of Late Deafened Adults (ALDA)
1027 Oakton
Evanston, IL 60202

Self Help for Hard of Hearing People (SHHH)
7910 Woodmont Ave., Suite 1200
Bethesda, MD 20814
301-657-2248

Public Information Sources

National Information Center on Deafness
Gallaudet University
800 Florida Ave, NE
Washington, DC 20002
202-651-5051

National Technical Institute for the Deaf
Resources Catalogue
PO Box 9887
Rochester, NY 14623-0887
716-475-6824

Chapter 5

Counseling Older Adults with Hearing Impairments

Samuel Trychin

I have been working with adults who are hard-of-hearing and their families for the past 8 years. These people have been participants in classes and workshops on the general topic of *Coping with Hearing Loss* (changed to *Living with Hearing Loss* because coping carries a negative connotation for some people). In this work I have seen more than 1000 people and have conducted programs in 43 states. Most people who have attended the sessions are older than 60 years.

Assumptions about older people who are hard-of-hearing relate to their apparent reluctance to take steps to deal with their hearing loss. One is that hearing loss is associated with "old age" and accepting the fact that one has hearing loss indicates that one has finally become "old." If people deny their hearing problems, they can delay being seen as or feeling old. Another assumption is that older people have difficulty changing the ways they do things and, therefore, resist using hearing aids and changing other aspects of their communication behavior.

We have no information to affirm or deny these allegations because the people with whom I work have come to us voluntarily (except for a few reluctant spouses who have been prodded to the sessions). Many have travelled hundreds of miles or more to attend the sessions and have been willing to spend the necessary time and money to learn about dealing with hearing loss. So, I simply do not see many people who deny their hearing loss; I see those who accept it and want to do something to deal with it.

There is a great commonality in the problem areas related to hearing loss reported by program participants, regardless of geographic location and age. For all those who have participated, communication difficulties and their psychologic and social effects rank as the most important concern. How this manifests itself is to some degree age-related. For example, communication problems related to work are not an issue for people who are retired from the work force. For younger people who are hard-of-hearing, problems may relate to getting a job; for older workers, problems may relate more to maintaining a job or advancing on the career ladder. For younger people with hearing losses, establishing relationships may be of paramount concern; for older people, maintaining existing relationships may be the issue. A few additional considerations related to age are as follows.

First, there seems to be an ethos among some people who came of age during the 1920s and 1930s that places high value on self-sufficiency. This may be because few community services were available at that time. This cultural-generational factor can make some older people uncomfortable with the idea of asking others to make changes to accommodate them or to go out of their way to include them. Such clients need to be assured that accommodations made to increase comprehension also benefit the speaker, who has to repeat less and feels less frustrated in communication.

Second, older people with hearing losses or other physical problems may be more concerned than younger people with hearing losses about maintaining independence. Some are concerned that they will develop a dependency on their hearing aid and that their remaining hearing will deteriorate as a result. Some may misinterpret requesting others to alter their communication behavior as a sign of increasing dependency. Such people need to see that efforts to cope with hearing loss, such as wearing hearing aids and informing others about how to best communicate, are necessary steps in maintaining or increasing independence.

Third, older people are more at risk of being isolated socially because of the death of a spouse or friends, because children have moved to a different state, or because of reduced opportunity to make new friends because of physical, financial, or other limitations. Some older people with hearing impairments live in virtual isolation—unable to use the telephone or television and seldom leaving their apartments or houses. Such people need help in acquiring and using assistive listening devices (ALDs) that enable them to use the telephone, watch television, and meet and talk to other people.

Fourth, among older people who have hearing losses, there is a greater likelihood that other physical problems may complicate their situation. For example, severe visual problems can preclude using speechreading or real-time captioning as supplements to hearing. Fine-motor coordination problems can interfere with operating the controls of a hearing aid or changing batteries when necessary.

Finally, a few much older people, very few, do not wish to do anything to compensate for their hearing loss because they have "heard it all before" and want to be left alone to be with their thoughts and memories. If possible, ruling out depression, anxiety, and related conditions may be in order to assure that the person is making the choice to "tune out" on the basis of a rational personal preference.

With the foregoing considerations in mind, I believe that the problems and solutions are similar for most people who have hearing losses and for those who interact with them, even though the settings within which the problems occur may vary with the age of the person. Additional age-related considerations are discussed later in the chapter.

LIVING WITH A HEARING-LOSS PROGRAM

Orientation

The program I have developed is educational rather than therapeutic in orientation in that it is a problem-solving approach that focuses on strategies for
preventing or reducing communication problems. The premise is that teaching people ways to prevent or reduce communication difficulties stemming
from a hearing loss is an effective method for resolving the psychologic and
social problems that result from such difficulties.

This approach operates on the assumption that either the speaker or the
listener or, more likely, both may experience problems when communication
breakdowns occur due to hearing loss. It is an interactional approach in that
it assumes that what the speaker does and says in response to a communication breakdown has an effect on the listener and vice versa; their reactions
influence what happens next between them. For example, if one or both become frustrated and irritated, the interaction will probably deteriorate in
some way. If they remain calm and relaxed, there is a better chance the two
will find a way to resolve the communication problem.

Goals

The goals of the program are as follows:

1. Raise participants' awareness of the situations that frequently produce
   communication difficulties for people with hearing losses and those
   with whom they communicate
2. Identify the causes of these communication problems
3. Identify the most frequently reported reactions to communication difficulties
4. Identify reactions that serve to increase the probability of occurrence of
   communication difficulties and specify how that occurs
5. Provide opportunity to practice alternative reactions—responses that
   serve to resolve communication problems when they occur
6. Provide opportunity to practice behavior that can prevent or reduce the
   occurrence of communication problems in the first place
7. Provide information about local and national resources

Program Content

The program provides information regarding hearing loss, ALDs, service
providers, and resources. It also provides the opportunity for participants to
learn and practice effective communication behavior that will prevent or reduce communication problems related to hearing loss and provide opportunity

for participants to identify and alter their dysfunctional responses to communication problems when they do occur. It is necessary to provide opportunity for participants to develop realistic, nonjudgmental attitudes toward hearing loss, those who have it, and those who relate to them.

Providing Correct Information

It is necessary to dispel several frequently encountered myths or misconceptions about hearing loss (Trychin, 1993). Some of these myths are as follows:

1. The hearing aid myth. The misconception is that hearing aids are the solution to all communication difficulties that stem from hearing loss. People think about hearing aids as being analogous to eyeglasses, that is, they restore hearing to normal. People need to learn that the benefits of hearing aids are situation-specific; they work well in some situations, less well in others, and poorly under other circumstances. Having realistic expectations about what hearing aids can do is one step toward increasing the use of aids and keeping them out of bureau drawers.
2. The speechreading myth. The misconception is that if one has a hearing loss, one is automatically a good speechreader. The fact is that not everyone can learn to be an effective speech reader. Visual problems, environmental variables, speaker factors, amount of residual hearing, and the large number of homophenous sounds (sounds that look alike, eg, /p/, /b/, and /m/) can determine how much information a person receives from speechreading alone.
3. The severity of loss determines the amount of handicap (disadvantage, functional limitation, disability, challenge) myth. An audiogram by itself is not a good index of the degree to which a person is handicapped by his or her hearing loss. One needs to know about the variety of listening situations a person encounters during the waking hours. It is necessary to determine the communication demands and the barriers to communication in each of those situations. Some people with severe or profound hearing losses work in situations that make no or few communication demands and are not handicapped on the job by their hearing loss. Some people with mild or moderate hearing losses may be in situations that make communication demands and present many barriers to communication. People need to know that communication situations vary in terms of demands and barriers and that understanding in one situation does not mean a person will understand in other situations.

It is necessary, as stated previously, to ensure that the participants receive correct, up-to-date information about hearing loss, hearing aids, ALDs, and local and national resources, including reading materials, appropriate professional services, and support groups.

Learning and Practicing Effective Communication
Behavior

Because listening situations vary considerably in terms of the communication demands on a listener and barriers to communication, it is important that participants learn to assess environments as they enter them and think about ways of overcoming potential problems. We try to train participants to assess each listening situation for possible barriers to communication. Examples of such barriers are background noise, poor lighting, and visual or other distractions (Trychin, 1991). Once the barriers are identified, the person should attempt to eliminate or reduce them or locate him- or herself to best advantage within the environment. This process is a first step in teaching participants to anticipate potential problems in situations and to plan strategies for preventing or reducing the problems.

It is important that participants have sufficient knowledge about ALDs and enough practice in their use to determine situations in which these devices can be used to advantage. When people learn to use appropriate devices in restaurants, meetings, parties, and automobiles, communication problems are frequently prevented or greatly reduced (Trychin & Albright, 1993). Practice with ALDs is often necessary for decreasing resistance to using them. Providing opportunity for participants to use ALDs outside the classroom, such as during lunch in a cafeteria, while conversing in a moving car, or at home watching television, can be effective in increasing the likelihood that the participant will consider purchasing and using the device.

Effective communication behavior involves the ability to identify aspects of communication behavior in oneself or in others that might contribute to communication problems. It also involves eliciting cooperation from others when there is need for others to change their behavior. People who are hard of hearing need to be able to perform the following functions:

1. Inform others about their hearing loss
2. Inform speakers about what to do to be understood
3. Politely remind others when they forget
4. Model the communication behavior they desire in others.

Speakers can do a number of things to increase the likelihood they will be understood. Examples are getting the listener's attention before beginning to talk, facing the listener, and speaking at a moderate pace (Trychin & Boone, 1987). Although it is true that these practices will improve understanding by any listener, they are imperative when talking to a person who is hard of hearing.

The speaker needs to know that the listener has a hearing loss and know what to do to be understood. It is usually the responsibility of the person with the hearing loss to inform speakers that they have a hearing loss and to inform them about what to do to be better understood. Many people who are hard-of-hearing state that they prefer to wait until there is an obvious communication problem before informing a speaker about their hearing loss. This strategy works well as long as the listener knows when he or she is not understanding what is being said. Problems develop with this strategy when the listener thought he or she understood but did not. If the listener gives no response, speakers cannot know whether or not they have been understood; they ordinarily assume they have been understood.

If the listener has misunderstood and makes an inappropriate response and the speaker does not know that there is a hearing problem, often the misunderstanding is attributed to another factor. That factor is frequently not very flattering, such as low intelligence, a personality problem, or lack of interest. The listener can minimize miscommunication by simply stating at the outset, "I have a hearing loss, and if I make an inappropriate response, you'll know it's because of that. If we have a communication problem, we can easily correct it." It usually requires some practice and support for participants to reach the point at which they feel comfortable about informing others about their hearing loss. It requires additional training and practice for participants to identify the causes of specific communication problems and state what needs to be changed to facilitate understanding (Trychin & Albright, 1993).

Misunderstanding may or may not be apparent to the speaker or the listener. A problem frequently reported by family members is that they are often unsure whether the person with the hearing loss has understood them or not. This results in needless repetition of words that have been heard and the erroneous assumption that speakers have been understood when they have not. If what has been said is not understood, but the speaker (and possibly the listener) does not know it, the consequences of the miscommunication may not be apparent until later. For example, a task is not done, a person arrives at the wrong place or time, the wrong person is contacted, or someone raises a topic that has just been discussed. This is one of the most important factors in weakening relationships and damaging self-esteem in that the person who is hard of hearing may come to be seen as, or come to see him- or herself as, being less than competent and dependable.

Relationship problems can develop when people who have hearing losses believe they have understood correctly when they have not. When a person is erroneously certain that he or she knows what has been said, arguments can ensue regarding what was and what was not said. It is even more of a problem if the person is not aware of having misunderstood someone such as a physician, attorney, or counselor. In these instances the misunderstood information can become firmly fixed in the person's mind; the person is certain, "My doctor told me . . . ."

It is important that people with hearing losses learn to repeat aloud the essentials of what they have heard. If something has been misunderstood, it can be quickly corrected. Important details such as who, what, when, and where especially need to be repeated by hard-of-hearing people so that speakers will know they have been understood.

Another issue is that many people who are hard-of-hearing bluff. Bluffing means pretending to understand when the person knows he or she did not understand what was said. Nodding and smiling as though one understands leads speakers to assume the message has been comprehended. It comes as an unpleasant shock to the speaker to learn later the listener really has not understood. Frequent reactions to this discovery are anger and resentment and the belief that the listener was simply not interested in what the speaker was saying. This is not a good way to nurture relationships. People with hearing losses need to learn to eliminate bluffing from their responses to communication problems. One of the main reasons that people bluff is that they do not know what else to do when they misunderstand someone. They need to learn about and use a variety of adaptive, alternative responses (Trychin, 1987; Trychin & Boone, 1987). This requires practice over time with feedback about how well the listener is doing and a great deal of encouragement.

Speakers need to be informed about what to do to be understood. Simple, descriptive, specific, and polite instructions get the best results. Such responses are, "I need to be able to see your face when you talk to me" or "Because of my hearing loss, I would appreciate it if you could slow down just a little." People who are hard-of-hearing need to learn to stop using expressions such as "Huh?" "What?" "Excuse me," "I'm sorry," "Would you repeat that?" "I didn't get that," and "I'm not following you." None of these responses provides information to speakers about what they need to do to be understood. All they do is indicate that there is a problem; they offer no solution and, therefore, waste time.

To be able to pinpoint the solutions to communication difficulties, the people involved have to know the causes of the difficulty. People are largely unaware of the variety of factors that operate to produce communication breakdowns. Most assume that communication problems are caused by hearing loss. A number of factors, however, cause or contribute to difficulty in understanding what is being said. I have found it helpful to organize the variety of causes of communication breakdowns under three categories of factors—speaker, environmental, and listener (Trychin, 1991). Table 5–1 lists a number of the causes of communication difficulties according to the three categories.

Family members benefit from a knowledge of the factors that contribute to communication problems. One of their most frequent complaints is, "I don't understand the variability in his (her) ability to follow what I'm saying. Sometimes, he (she) understands everything I say and, other times, nothing. I think he (she) can understand me when he (she) wants to." The latter statement invariably leads to an argument. Knowing the factors that influence understanding removes the mystery from the situation for family members. They then realize that people with hearing losses are more likely to understand better in the morning when they are well rested than later in the day, better in the quiet of the living room than in a noisy kitchen, and better when they are able to see the speaker's face than when they cannot.

TABLE 5–1 Sources of Communication Difficulties for Adults with Hearing Impairments

SPEAKER CAUSES PROBLEM

Talks too rapidly

Talks too softly (or loudly)

Speech is not clear

Does not first get listener's attention

Is too far away to be heard

Has hands or objects obscuring face

Talks from another room or from behind listener

Is obviously annoyed, irritated, or angry

Talks while person with hearing impairment is involved in another activity

Turns face away from listener while talking

Drops voice at end of sentence

ENVIRONMENT CAUSES PROBLEM

Several people speaking and conversation flows rapidly back and forth between them

Interfering background noise

Poor illumination

Obstacles prevent listener from seeing speaker's face

Distractions are present

Room acoustics are poor

Room ventilation is poor

Message is coming over a public address system

LISTENER IS CAUSE OF PROBLEM

Does not pay attention (eg, is distracted by thoughts, sensations, or tinnitus) or is not motivated to hear

Uses hearing aid inefficiently

Is tired

Is emotionally upset (eg, anxious, angry, or depressed)

Has poor speechreading skills

Is not using assistive listening devices

Has low expectations about what can be understood in the situation

Has a hearing loss so severe it prevents understanding

Has a speech discrimination deficit that prevents understanding

Has visual problems that interfere with seeing the speaker's face

Does not inform speaker about not understanding

Does not inform speaker about how to communicate effectively

Effective communication behavior involves dealing with other people's forgetting to communicate properly. It is important that people who have hearing losses understand that other people will forget, and forget frequently, about the hearing loss. Because hearing loss is an invisible handicap even those who live with a hard-of-hearing person forget to alter their communication behavior to be understood. They speak from another room, speak too rapidly, and speak too softly. When reminded, they change their behavior for a while and then revert back to their previous behavior. This occurs because people are much more interested in what they are saying than in how they are saying it; it is not because they are insensitive, mean, or uncaring. Furthermore, changing our overlearned, habitual, and unconscious communication behavior is difficult and often requires special procedures (Trychin & Albright, 1993). When people who have hearing losses recognize these facts and the fact that they themselves often forget and communicate in ineffective ways, their anger and resentment toward family members who forget is greatly diminished.

Finally, an effective way to help others adopt facilitative communication behavior is to model the desired behavior. If I want you to stop talking to me from another room, I had better practice coming to where you are when I want to tell you something. People with hearing losses should demonstrate the rate and loudness of speech they desire in others by talking at that rate and loudness themselves.

Identifying and Altering Dysfunctional Responses

In addition to the communication behaviors discussed previously, other factors interfere with understanding and can be destructive to relationships. Dominating conversations is one example. Withdrawing by staying home or by not participating in conversations is another example of behaviors that do not promote meaningful interaction.

Negative emotional reactions to communication problems, such as anger, depression, anxiety, and guilt, interfere with understanding and often alienate other people. Thought disturbances that result from communication difficulties, such as excessive worrying, inability to think clearly, and inability to focus attention on a speaker, interfere with following a speaker and interfere with finding solutions to communication problems. Physical reactions such as headaches, painful muscle tension, and stomach pain or nausea, are distractions that compete for the sufferer's attention and make it difficult to focus on what a speaker is saying (Trychin, 1991). It is important that people become able to identify these reactions and replace them with others that promote, rather than interfere with, understanding. Providing people with homework assignments that help them identify their reactions when communication problems develop and giving them opportunity to practice constructive responses in the safety of the class situation are effective methods for reducing the frequency of dysfunctional responses. Examples of such exercises are contained in Trychin and Albright (1993).

Developing Realistic, Nonjudgmental Attitudes

One of the more important outcomes of the workshops and classes is a change in the attitude of many participants. There often is a reduction in negative, judgmental valuation of others and of the participants. This effect is probably brought about by the information the participants receive from the instructor and from the other fellow participants. Family members and friends are able to hear the perspectives of a variety of people who have hearing losses, and people with hearing losses learn about what life is like for the people with normal hearing who frequently interact with people who have hearing losses. It is important that people hear the other side from someone other than their spouse, parent, or child. It seems easier to hear what someone is saying when that person is further removed personally.

Becoming skilled in communication practices that prevent or reduce communication problems allows participants to become relaxed in social situations and to feel better about themselves. Eliminating tension and experiencing enjoyment in social situations seems to have a positive influence on the person's general attitude.

Using Support Groups as Resources

It is to the advantage of people who have hearing losses and their family members to belong to and attend support group meetings in which members share common experiences and concerns. Self Help for Hard of Hearing People (SHHH), for example, is a national organization with more than 150 local chapters throughout the United States. SHHH is unrivaled for the information and support it provides to thousands of people who are hard-of-hearing. Hundreds of SHHH members have told my associates and me about the benefits they have derived from their membership.

STRUCTURE OF THE LIVING-WITH-HEARING-LOSS PROGRAM

Format for Classes

A group format is used exclusively because my experience indicates that positive changes in communication behavior occur more rapidly in a group than in individuals or couples counseling. To emphasize the educational focus, I use the term *class* rather than *group*. The number of participants per class is limited to 12 to provide each person with sufficient individual attention. Classes are conducted in one of two time frames. In the first, participants meet once a week in 2- to 3-hour sessions for 12 to 15 weeks. In the second time frame, participants meet 6 to 8 hours a day for 5 to 7 days. In either format it is best to have people attend for about 40 hours to cover most of the material related to preventing or reducing communication problems and to provide sufficient time for participants to practice the procedures and techniques suggested in the class.

The group format provides opportunity to observe each participant's communication behavior. Rather than lecturing, the group facilitator asks questions to elicit suggestions and information from participants and to witness their communication behavior. When appropriate communication behavior occurs, it is brought to the group's attention and rewarded (I use play money). When they are made, for example, a person does not pay attention to a speaker, communication errors are immediately brought to the person's attention and corrections promptly suggested and practiced. In this process it is imperative to use humor (we use a rubber doll whose eyes, ears, and nose pop out when the doll is squeezed) and other strategies that reduce the likelihood that participants will feel criticized and become defensive.

Format for Workshops

Workshops usually take place on weekends in one of two formats. The first is 1-day sessions (6 hours) that accommodate up to 100 people. These sessions are mostly lectures with some discussion, depending on the number of participants. The more people in the class, the less discussion there is because of the logistical problems in having everyone understand. The second workshop format is 2-day sessions limited to 25 people in which more time is devoted to discussion among the participants.

No matter what the format, it is important to schedule breaks at least every hour when there are people with hearing losses in the session. Sustained visual attention is quite fatiguing for them, and they experience difficulty paying attention for long periods of time.

Age-Related Considerations

When participants are old or frail, session lengths are limited to an hour and a half with a break about half-way through. Judgment must be used about how far to press an older person in terms of changing his or her communication behavior. For some older people, it may be appropriate to focus on ALDs that will help them better understand what is said on the television or over the telephone. Introducing elderly people to alerting devices that increase their sense of safety and security may be all that can be done in some cases. Usually, if the person is healthy and active with a desire to maintain relationships with friends and family, he or she will be interested in the variety of communication issues discussed previously. In any event, one cannot exceed what each person is willing to accept and do. Instructors can elicit suggestions for resolving problems and suggest some of their own, but it is up to each participant to try the suggestions.

I have conducted classes in eight different senior centers. Some participants attended the centers routinely every day, and others came in from the community only for the classes. My impression was that the participants who came specifically for the classes received more benefit than those who routinely attended the centers. One reason is that many of those who visited the centers on a daily basis tended to be frailer and less independent—many were brought to the centers by family members. Another possible reason is that people who visit the centers on a regular basis may see such programs as entertainment rather than education. In many centers, entertainment activities are scheduled throughout the day, and it is possible that almost any program may be perceived as entertainment by regular visitors. In two centers with more affluent and more highly educated attendees, the entertainment factor was not a problem.

I conducted auditory screenings of approximately 200 older people (mean age about 65 years) in three different locations. I referred about 50 percent of the people screened for further evaluation by an audiologist or for medical treatment. In one senior center, eight of the people who came for the screening already had hearing aids. The audiologist who was conducting the screenings determined that seven of the eight hearing aids were in need of repair.

These experiences indicated that there is a need to find ways to deliver services to older people who are hard-of-hearing and that outreach efforts by audiologists need to be greatly expanded because many older people with hearing losses are unable or unwilling to go to where the services are ordinarily provided. These older people may be experiencing other family or medical problems that are assigned higher priority for immediate attention. Many older people with hearing losses do not have the money or transportation needed to obtain audiologic services, especially if they reside in rural or suburban areas. Others are simply unaware that there is anything that can be done to compensate for the hearing loss. Some elders have been told by their family physician or other professional that "There is nothing you can do about it; you'll just have to learn to live with it."

My experience also indicated that audiologic services need to be expanded to include the issues discussed previously in this chapter. For many people who have hearing losses, wearing a hearing aid is only part of the solution to communication problems and their psychosocial effects. Identifying and changing environmental barriers, eliciting appropriate speaker behavior, and adopting effective listener behavior are necessary for living with a hearing loss.

REFERENCES

Trychin, S. (1987). *Did I do that?* Washington: Gallaudet University.

Trychin, S. (1991). *Manual for mental health professionals. II. Psychosocial challenges faced by hard of hearing people.* Washington: Gallaudet University.

Trychin, S. (1993). *Communication issues related to hearing loss.* Washington: Gallaudet University.

Trychin, S. & Albright, J. (1993). *Staying in touch.* Washington: Gallaudet University.

Trychin, S., & Boone, M. (1987). *Communication rules for hard of hearing people.* Washington: Gallaudet University.

SUGGESTED READING

Bally, S., & Trychin, S. (Eds.) (1989). *A newcomer's guide to an old problem: Hearing loss.* Washington: Gallaudet University.

Forgatch, M., & Trychin, S. (1988). *Getting along* [manual]. Washington: Gallaudet University.

Forgatch, M., & Trychin, S. (1988). *Getting along* [videotape]. Washington: Gallaudet University.

Trychin, S. (1986). *Relaxation training for hard of hearing people: Audiotapes.* Washington: Gallaudet University.

Trychin, S. (1986). *Relaxation training for hard of hearing people: Trainee's manual.* Washington: Gallaudet University.

Trychin, S. (1986). *Relaxation training for hard of hearing people: Videotapes.* Washington: Gallaudet University.

Trychin, S. (1986). *Stress management video series for deaf people: Trainee's manual.* Washington: Gallaudet University.

Trychin, S. (1986). *Stress management video series for deaf people: Videotapes.* Washington: Gallaudet University.

Trychin, S. (1987). *Communication rules for hard of hearing people* [videotape]. Washington: Gallaudet University.

Trychin, S. (1987). Did I do that? [videotape]. Washington: Gallaudet University.

Trychin, S. (1987). *Relaxation training for hard of hearing people: Practitioner's manual.* Washington: Gallaudet University.

Trychin, S. (1987). *Stress management video series for deaf people: Practitioner's manual.* Washington: Gallaudet University.

Trychin, S. (1988). *So THAT'S the Problem!.* Washington: Gallaudet University.

Trychin, S. (1990). *Speak out: Tips on speaking in public for individuals with a hearing loss.* Washington: Gallaudet University.

Trychin, S., & Bonvillian, B. (1991). *Actions speak louder: Tips for putting on skits relating to hearing loss.* Washington: Gallaudet University.

Trychin, S., & Boone, M. (1987). *Communication rules for hard of hearing people: Manual.* Washington: Gallaudet University.

Trychin, S., & Busacco, D. (1991). *Manual for mental health professionals. I. Making services accessible to hard of hearing people.* Washington: Gallaudet University.

Trychin, S., & Wright, F. (1988). *Is THAT What You Think?* Washington: Gallaudet University.

Chapter 6

Beyond Hearing Aids: Use of Auxiliary Aids

Sharon A. Sandridge

For most people with presbycusic hearing losses, amplification is invaluable. But even the best hearing aid can not solve all the problems a person may have. Hearing aids perform optimally when users are in a quiet environment in a one-to-one situation. As the primary signal becomes degraded through the introduction of increased distance, poor room acoustics, or the presence of a competing signal, the performance of the hearing aid is compromised. Communication, however, is not usually confined to quiet one-to-one situations. Communication includes dinner for two at a busy restaurant, gatherings of friends to watch a football game on television, attending a play or a movie, bowling, and attending religious services, conferences, or lecture series. All these situations involve less-than-ideal listening situations that may limit the performance of a hearing aid.

With an assistive listening device (ALD), distance can be decreased, signal-to-noise ratio (S/N) improved, and room acoustics minimized. By coupling a hearing aid to an ALD or replacing the hearing aid with an ALD, performance in less-than-optimal listening situations can be improved.

Communication is not the only event that may be compromised by a hearing loss. Ramsdell (1966) suggested that hearing operates on three levels: background, warning, and symbolic. The sense of hearing allows us to hear background sounds and remain in touch with the environment—the birds singing, the hum of the car. The sense of hearing is also the primary mode for warning—sirens announcing an approaching emergency vehicle, a car horn warning one not to step off the curb. Hearing at both these levels can be compromised by a hearing loss, and both are reasons to wear amplification. Yet, hearing-aid performance may be limited in these areas. And hearing aids are not worn 24 hours a day, which results in a reduction of the audibility of background and warning sounds, such as smoke alarms and doorbells.

The ability to hear background sounds and warning signals fosters a sense of security and independence. This security can be maintained with alerting devices. Devices that alert one to the presence of a knock on the door or the smoke alarm assist in maintaining the awareness of background sounds and warning signals.

When dealing with older adults, hearing care professionals should try to ascertain any and all problems, difficulties, and concerns that may exist because of the presence of a hearing loss. Hearing care professionals must go beyond dispensing hearing aids as if the aids meet patients' needs for communication, background awareness, and warning. Listening situations that cause difficulty must be fully assessed, and solutions to reduce the handicapping nature of the hearing loss must be provided. ALDs must be used as routinely as hearing aids.

The purpose of this chapter is to present ways to solve problems that exist because of the presence of a hearing loss and to become full-service hearing care providers. The intent is to provide a practical clinical approach to implementing ALDs and alerting devices into the daily provision of services for clients to provide them with the most comprehensive care possible.

TERMINOLOGY

The terms *assistive listening device* (ALD) and *alerting device* have been the descriptive terms for devices used by audiologists. Although the terms *assistive listening device* and *alerting device* are descriptive in nature and categorical, they are restrictive. For example, real-time captioning is considered an ALD, but it does not actually assist in listening; it assists by presenting an aural message visually. The term *auxiliary aid*, on the other hand, is nonrestrictive and noncategorical. Any device that provides additional assistance is considered an auxiliary aid. Auxiliary aids include frequency modulation (FM) systems, amplified telephone handsets, smoke detectors, closed captioning, and real-time captioning devices. Note takers, sign-language interpreters, and oral interpreters provide auxiliary services. The assistance can be delivered in the auditory, visual, or tactile mode. It can alert one to the presence of a signal, enhance the audibility of a signal, or facilitate communication by presenting the aural signal in a visual mode. Auxiliary aids encompass any and all devices that promote effective communication.

SELECTION OF AUXILIARY AIDS

When considering an auxiliary aid or device, the following three questions must be asked (Figure 6–1):

1. How will the signal be picked up?
2. How will the signal be transmitted?
3. How will the signal be delivered?

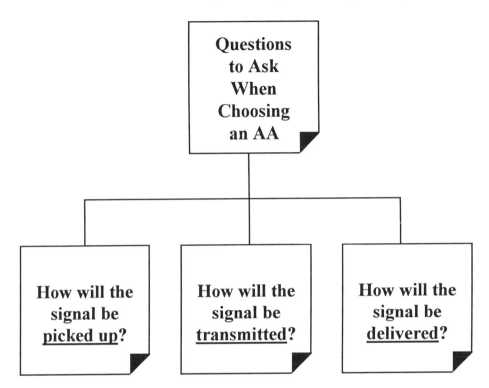

FIGURE 6–1 *Three questions that should be asked in selecting listening or alerting devices.*

How Will The Signal Be Picked Up?

One of three methods can be used for signal pickup—a microphone, direct connection, or induction (Table 6–1).

TABLE 6–1 How the Signal Is Picked Up

MICROPHONE
Most flexible and adaptable
Different microphones can be used for different situations
Need to consider size, power, frequency response, physical design, polarity, impedance, connecting cable length
DIRECT CONNECTION
Plugs directly into an audio-out plug
Provides good fidelity
Can bypass external speaker
Works best with telephones, radios, televisions, doorbells

TABLE 6–1 How the Signal Is Picked Up (continued)

INDUCTION PICKUP
Picks up electromagnetic energy
May be susceptible to outside interference
Works primarily with telephones or doorbells

Microphone

The most common input device is the microphone. It is easily adapted to most situations. By simply placing a microphone near any sound source, at any location, for any device, the signal can be picked up. All microphones serve the same function—to pick up an acoustic signal and transduce it into electrical energy; yet all microphones are not the same. They differ in the size of the pickup area, power, frequency response, physical design, polarity, impedance, and power supply needed. In addition, some microphones are affected by changes in the length of the connecting cord or the presence of outside interference. When choosing a microphone, especially for situations that involve speech, the user must consider these factors to maximize reception.

In addition, the most appropriate microphone for a given situation may not be the microphone originally supplied with a device, especially if speech is the input. The user should not limit the performance of a device by using a less than appropriate microphone. Experimentation is required. It is advisable to have several microphones that range in size, directionality, impedance, and type available for trial. Microphones are available from distributors of ALDs, some hearing-aid manufacturers, or the local electronics store.

Direct Connection

Some auxiliary aids can be connected directly to the sound source with a plug or jack connection or can be wired into the main electrical system. When the plug from the transmitting device (eg, the AudioLink Infrared System) is inserted into the audio-out jack (eg, of a television), the signal is transferred directly. This connection reduces the risk of distortion during acoustic to electrical transduction and provides a high-fidelity signal. The installation is easy; it involves the simple attachment of the male plug from the transmitting device into the female audio-out receptor on the television or radio.

One potential disadvantage of using the audio-out jack is that the external speaker may be turned off when the plug is inserted. Some televisions and radios are designed to disconnect the external speaker when the audio input is connected. In addition, many televisions and radios are not equipped with audio-out connections, thereby eliminating direct connection as a possibility for signal pickup.

Direct connection can also be used with telephones and doorbells. Many telephone alerting devices connect directly into the modular phone jack. If a phone jack is not available, any jack can be adapted to accommodate more than one phone plug by using an outlet adapter (available from telephone stores, electronics stores, or auxillary aid distributors). This allows the telephone line and the line from the auxiliary aid to be connected in the same jack. When the electrical impulse signals the telephone to ring, it also activates the auxiliary aid, such as a phone alerting device.

The third possible direct connection is wiring the device directly into the existing electrical system. Doorbell auxiliary aids, for example, can be connected directly to the wiring of the existing doorbell. This type of direct connection is slightly more involved than other direct connection methods and may require an electrician. This type of installation also tends to be permanent.

Induction Pickup

The third option for signal pickup is induction. Induction pickup requires the presence of electromagnetic energy, so it is limited primarily to telephones and doorbells. Because this type of pickup is restricted to electromagnetic energy, it is not as susceptible to outside acoustic interference. For example, if an alerting device is needed for telephone use in a busy office, a microphone is contraindicated because the microphone picks up any acoustic event (eg, anyone talking around the microphone). The use of direct connection is contraindicated because of physical restrictions (ie, location and the wiring of the telephone system). An induction pickup device, therefore, is the most appropriate option. The alerting device is activated only when electromagnetic energy is generated by the ringer of the telephone. One disadvantage is that many modern telephones no longer use electromagnetic ringers.

How Will the Signal Be Transmitted?

Signal transmission can occur by four methods—direct connection (hardwired); frequency modulated radio waves (FM systems); infrared light waves (infrared systems); and electromagnetic energy (induction loop systems). Each method (Table 6–2) or system offers advantages and disadvantages. In many cases there is not a clear advantage of one system over the other systems. In other cases, only one system is the most appropriate. It is important to keep in mind that a system appropriate for all situations does not exist.

Hard-Wired Systems

A hard-wired system uses a direct electrical connection in the delivery of the signal. Figure 6–2 illustrates such a system. Hard-wired systems typically

TABLE 6–2 How the Signal Is Transmitted

WIRED SYSTEMS
Hard-wired

WIRELESS SYSTEMS
Frequency modulation systems

Infrared systems

Induction loop systems

involve a connection (ie, a cord or cords) between the input device (ie, microphone), a transmitter (eg, PockeTalker), and an output device (ie, earphones). Hard-wired systems (Table 6–3) are generally the least expensive of the four systems, yet they provide excellent sound transmission and quality. They are also portable and adaptable.

Hard-wired systems are most applicable in situations in which mobility is not needed. Because the use of long cords may present a safety hazard, hard-wired systems are generally not applicable for large-group listening situations. Another disadvantage of a hard-wired system is its lack of compatibility with other assistive listening systems. With the implementation of the Americans with Disabilities Act (ADA), many theaters, cinemas, and concert halls are installing wireless assistive listening systems that are not compatible with individual hard-wired systems.

A number of hard-wired systems are available, ranging from inexpensive units, such as the Whisper 2000, to the moderately priced Williams Sound

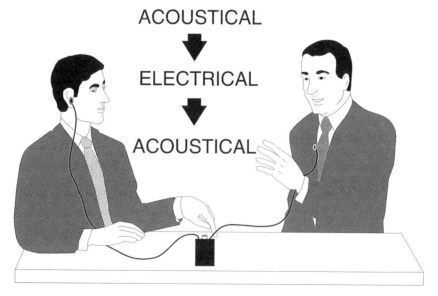

FIGURE 6–2 *A hard-wired system such as a PockeTalker. The talker and the listener are tethered to each other. Best situations are one-to-one in which mobility is not an issue.*

TABLE 6–3 Hard-wired Systems

SUMMARY

Uses a direct electrical connection between sender and receiver

A cord connects the entire system

Excellent signal transmission and quality

ADVANTAGES

Least expensive system

Portable and adaptable

Good for one-to-one or small-group listening situations

Generally excellent sound quality

DISADVANTAGES

Tethered to the source

Lack of mobility

Not compatible with any other listening system

PockeTalker, to more expensive auditory trainers. Dempsey and Ross (1994) conducted a subjective and an objective evaluation of six hard-wired systems used by a group of 18 adults with hearing impairments. The frequency response when the systems were coupled to KEMAR (Knowles Electronics Manikin for Acoustic Research) along with subjective measurements of speech understanding, sound quality, and ease of use were evaluated. The frequency response was found to be substantially different for each of the six devices tested. Subjective ratings for speech understanding and sound quality were also found to differ among the devices. When rated for ease of use, performance was comparable for the least and most expensive devices and best for the moderately priced devices.

It would seem prudent, then, not to make the assumption that every device is comparable and that price is directly related to performance. Assessment of the frequency response of each device and a trial period should be offered (Dempsey, 1994; Palmer, 1992) when an audiologist recommends and fits any auxiliary aid.

An example of how the device can be used in a number of situations without concern about installation, interference, and other factors follows.

Mrs. Nan is an older woman who has a hearing loss and wears binaural in-the-ear (ITE) hearing aids. One of the hearing aids has a telecoil. Mrs. Nan has been relatively satisfied and pleased with her amplification but is having difficulty in a particular situation. She drives her three friends and herself to their weekly bridge game. She has found that it is extremely difficult to follow the conversation among the women in the car. Because of the road and car noise and because she is driving, Mrs. Nan cannot speechread.

After assessing the situation, Mrs. Nan and her audiologist decided to try a PockeTalker personal amplification system (Williams Sound, Eden

Prairie, MN) coupled to a neckloop. This system would enable Mrs. Nan to pick up her friends' voices at a greater signal-to-noise ratio through the telecoil while still being able to hear the road noises and warning signals through the other hearing aid. The microphone for the Pocketalker was placed in the middle on top of the back of the front seat. A small piece of hook-and-loop fastener was placed on the seat to keep the microphone in place. This system allows anyone in the car to use the microphone, such as Mrs. Don. Mrs. Nan had extra difficulty hearing Mrs. Don because Mrs. Don has a soft voice. With the new system, when Mrs. Don wishes to talk, she removes the microphone from its position on the seat and places it in front of her mouth. When she is finished, she replaces the microphone. The other passengers are now requesting a Pocketalker to hear Mrs. Don.

Orienting her friends to the use of the microphone required several gentle reminders, but in less than a month and with less than a $200.00 investment, Mrs. Nan was able to continue as an active participant in the pre-bridge conversation. The system allowed the four women to maintain a social activity that brought great pleasure to them but was being compromised by Mrs. Nan's hearing loss. Mrs. Nan also uses the PockeTalker during the bridge game to make sure she hears the bids.

FM Systems

FM systems use radio waves rather than direct electrical connection to transmit a signal. No cords connect the transmitter and the receiver, so the listener is not tethered to the talker or the input signal (Figure 6–3, Table 6–4).

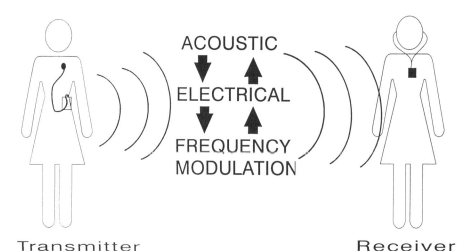

FIGURE 6–3 *FM system transmission.*

TABLE 6–4 FM Systems

SUMMARY

Uses radio frequencies to transmit signals

40 narrowband (NB) frequencies. Most common NB frequency is channel 26, 72.9 MHz

10 wideband (WB) frequencies. Most common WB frequency is channel E

ADVANTAGES

Can be used indoors or outdoors

Direct line-of-sight to transmitter not needed

No dead spots in listening area

No limit on number of receivers that can be used

Receivers can be individually tuned

Easy to install

Complete mobility

DISADVANTAGES

Privacy is difficult to maintain

Susceptible to interference from other FM systems, cordless telephones, beeper systems, large sheets of metal

Cost is higher than induction loop and hard-wired systems

Inconsistent electroacoustic performance (variability across units)

The acoustic signal, in general, is picked up by a microphone and converted to an electrical signal. This electrical signal is carried to the transmitter by a hard-wired connection. The transmitter transduces the electrical signal into a FM signal, which is then transmitted by a radio-frequency carrier wave to a receiver. The receiver picks up the radio transmission, demodulates the signal, amplifies the signal (filtering may also occur), and sends it to the output device (eg, earphones or neckloop), which transduces the signal into an audible signal.

The Federal Communications Commission (FCC) has allocated 40 NB and 10 WB channels for general hearing assistance. The 40 NB channels, designated by the numbers 1 through 40, range from 72.025 to 77.975 MHz and are separated by 50 kHz. NB channels are most commonly found in auditory trainers and personal FM systems or in situations in which a number of FM units broadcast simultaneously within a restricted area.

WB channels are designated by the letters A through J and are separated by 200 kHz. The WB channels are used for large-group listening situations, such as concert halls, auditoriums, and theaters, in which there is need for fewer channels and a greater dynamic range.

It is important to note that WB and NB systems are not compatible with each other. A NB receiver may not be able to detect the bandwidth from a WB transmitter; likewise, a WB receiver may not be able to receive a NB transmission with the same clarity and fidelity as a compatible receiver. For this reason it is imperative that the bandwidth and the frequency channel be known if there are plans to use a personal receiver with other FM systems. For example, the Extend-Ear (AVR Sonovation, Chanhassen, MN), a FM system housed in a behind-the-ear (BTE) hearing aid, uses a WB system, so it is not compatible with Phonic Ear (Phonic Ear, Petaluma, CA) or Telex (Telex Communications, Inc., Minneapolis, MN) NB FM auditory systems. The Phonic Ear FreeEar BTE-FM system (Phonic Ear, Petaluma, CA), however, is a NB system and fully compatible with all the NB Phonic Ear FM auditory trainers and wide-area listening systems.

Although the band of frequencies from 72 to 76 MHz is designated for hearing assistance, it is not a restricted band. FM systems have to share the air waves with pocket pagers, rural telephone transmitters, call boxes for emergency services, and portable communication systems, among others, all of which are licensed devices. There is a national movement, however, to have the FCC restrict the 72- to 76-MHz frequency bands for sole use by people with hearing impairments, which should assist in the reduction of interference.

Infrared Systems

The second wireless system is the infrared system (Figure 6–4, Table 6–5). This system uses harmless, invisible, infrared light waves that are just outside the boundaries of visible light. It is a slightly more complicated system than the other three systems, involving more components and requiring greater power, yet it is popular and quite effective.

Signal transmitted via light waves

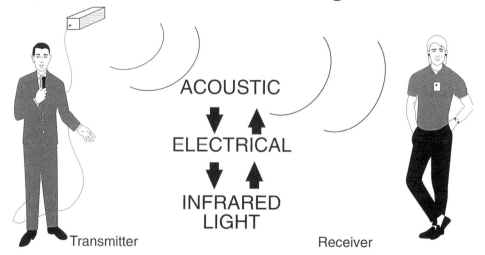

FIGURE 6–4 Infrared system transmission.

TABLE 6–5 Infrared Systems

SUMMARY

Transmits via invisible, infrared light waves

Infrared light waves travel in straight line

Absorbed by dark objects; reflected by shiny objects

Transmitters can be monophonic or multichannel

More diodes—more powerful signal—greater distance

Each diode has a 30- to 50-foot range

ADVANTAGES

No spillover

Privacy and confidentially maintained

Easy to use and install

Receiver compatible with most other transmitters

Different types of receivers and coupling options

DISADVANTAGES

Installation is more complicated than other systems

Cost higher than other three systems

Use limited to areas with little or no natural sunlight

Receivers less adjustable than FM receivers

Like the FM system, the infrared system consists of a transmitter and a receiver. In addition, it consists of a radiator or emitter and cables to connect the transmitter to the radiator. Infrared systems require too much power to be battery operated so an alternating current (AC) power source is needed, even in small personal systems.

The electrical signal, from either the microphone or direct connection, travels to the transmitter for modulation before conversion to infrared waves. Although several methods exist to modulate the signal, the most common procedure is through the frequency modulation of the signal on a carrier frequency. The transmitter can be monophonic or multichannel. The monophonic transmitter is the most common and transmits only one light-wave frequency. The most common carrier frequency is 95 kHz. Because of this standard carrier frequency, almost any receiver is compatible with any infrared transmitter. The multichannel transmitter can transmit multiple frequencies. An example of an infrared system with a multichannel transmitter is the system used at the United Nations to transmit simultaneous translation of different languages. Several receivers now offer two channels: 95 kHz and 250 kHz.

From the transmitter, the signal is converted to infrared light by the radiator or emitter. Radiators contain light-emitting diodes (LEDs), which emit light with a wavelength of 930 nM. The radiators are powered by the transmitter. If the system is a personal unit, the radiator and transmitter are housed in one unit. If the system is for large-area or large-group listening, the units are separate and must be connected by cables. It is possible to couple several radiators to one transmitter for large listening areas.

Receivers contain photodiodes that operate in the reverse of the LEDs by converting the infrared light into electrical signals. Infrared light travels in a straight line. It does not bend around corners or go through walls. If an object is in the path of the light, a shadow is cast and interference occurs, or the signal is eliminated. The best possible transmission occurs when there is a direct line of sight between the radiator and the receiving diodes. To ensure that a direct line of sight is maintained, several radiators may have to be installed in large listening areas such as auditoriums or theaters. For optimal signal transmission, the radiators should be placed as high as possible, in the upper corners of the room, tilting downward. For one-to-one use, the transmitter should be in direct line of sight.

Infrared light is absorbed by dark or dull surfaces and reflected by light or shiny surfaces. The absorption of infrared light limits the use of an infrared system to rooms that do not have windows or shiny reflecting walls. It is this absorption, however, that allows the isolation of the infrared signal. By hanging opaque curtains higher than the transmitter and radiator, a room can be partitioned into smaller listening areas, creating several independent transmitting areas without fear of interference from neighboring systems.

Induction Loops

The induction loop (Figure 6–5, Table 6–6) is the oldest of the wireless systems; it has been in existence for more than 40 years. The system is based on the principle of electromagnetic induction first described by Faraday in 1831 (Veley & Dulin, 1983).

TABLE 6–6 Induction Loop Systems

SUMMARY

Oldest of the wireless systems

Based on the principle of electromagnetic induction

Any size listening area can be looped

The greater the area, the more power is needed

No special receivers needed

Efficiency depends on strength of field and performance of the induction coil

ADVANTAGES

No receivers to maintain

Least expensive system

Installation is relatively easy

Maintenance is minimal

Spillover possible

Signal transmitted via electromagnetic waves

Hearing Aid
on "T"

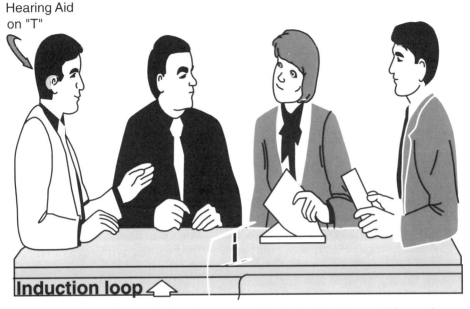

Induction loop

FIGURE 6–5 *Use of an induction loop system. A wire is placed around the conference table, allowing use of the hearing-aid telecoil. A small microphone is placed on the table facing the farthest talkers to facilitate ease of listening.*

TABLE 6–6 Induction Loop Systems (continued)

Quality depends on performance of telecoil or induction coil

Strength of electromagnetic field varies

Dead spots occur

Portability is limited

Susceptible to electromagnetic interference

DISADVANTAGES

In the audio induction loop system, the microphone receives the acoustic signal and converts it into an electrical current. The electrical current is passed through an amplifier and then sent through a wire that encircles a chair, a table, a room, or the neck of a person. This current sets up an electromagnetic field. If a telecoil circuit is placed close to the looped wire, an identical electrical current, which replicates the frequency and intensity of the signal from the loop, is induced. This electrical energy is conducted to the hearing-aid receiver, which converts the energy to an acoustic signal.

The induction loop system consists of an input device, an amplifier, and a transmitting device, which is the loop of wire. The input device is typically a microphone. However, for settings in which a public address system already exists, it is efficient to use direct connection to the public address system rather than to provide a separate microphone. An amplifier is necessary to boost the signal.

The third component, the transmitting loop of wire, can be any size or shape. The perimeter of any room can be looped (the longer the wire, the more power is needed). The loop can be permanently installed or it can be portable. For permanent installations, the loop is usually placed under the carpet or around the baseboard. If that is not feasible, the loop can be placed on the ceiling for use in the room above it. Sections of the room rather than the entire room can be looped.

It is also possible to loop smaller areas, such as the bottom of a conference table for small-group listening situations, the chair where a person sits to watch television, or even the neck of a person. The smallest field is that of a silhouette inductor, a small, thin, device in the shape of a BTE hearing aid that sits behind the ear and emits an electromagnetic field.

Missing from this system, compared with the other wireless systems, is the need for special receivers. One advantage of the induction loop system is that, in theory, anyone wearing a hearing aid with a telecoil can use the system simply by engaging the telecoil. Receivers are available, however, if a hearing aid is not equipped with a telecoil. These receivers range in size from that of a FM receiver to that of an in-the-canal (ITC) hearing aid. It has been estimated that less than 30 percent of hearing aids are equipped with telecoils (Stone, 1993), therefore 70 percent of hearing aid users cannot use the induction loop systems without special receivers.

How Will the Signal Be Delivered to the User?

Once a signal has been picked up and transmitted, it must be delivered, either through an enhanced auditory mode or conversion into a visual or tactile mode (Table 6–7). The choice depends on the situation (alerting or communicating), the degree of hearing with and without amplification, and personal preference. If the user has enough hearing with and without amplification, the auditory mode may be the most appropriate method. If the user is deaf or functionally deaf without hearing aids, a visual signal or a tactile signal may be more appropriate.

Auditory Mode

Delivery of the signal through an enhanced auditory mode is, perhaps, the easiest and most common method. The signal can be delivered in a number of ways (Figure 6–6): through a speaker with or without hearing aids; through earphones or earbuds; through hearing aids by direct audio input (DAI) or induction loop, silhouette, or induction receiver.

TABLE 6–7 How the Signal Is Delivered

Mode	Example
Auditory	Loudspeaker
	Headphones, earphones
	Direct audio input (DAI)
	Inductive coupling
Visual	Captioning—real, open, closed
	Computer modem
	Facsimile
	Lights
Tactile	Fans
	Vibrators
	Hearing dogs

The performance of each device is not equivalent. A number of studies have investigated the performance of different receivers when coupled to an FM system. In general, the frequency response from DAI showed a reduction for the low frequencies and either reduced or enhanced response for the high frequencies (Hawkins & Schum, 1985; Hawkins & Van Tasell, 1982; Thibodeau, 1990) along with an increase in equivalent noise (Hawkins & Van Tasell, 1982; Thibodeau, 1990). Reductions by as much as 18 dB across the frequency response were found when a neckloop was used (Hawkins & Van Tasell, 1982; Hawkins & Schum, 1985; Thibodeau et al. 1988; Thibodeau &

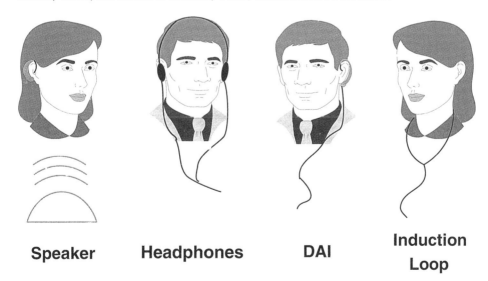

Speaker   **Headphones**   **DAI**   **Induction Loop**

FIGURE 6–6 *Options for delivering the signal by way of the auditory modality.*

Saucedo, 1991; Van Tasell & Landin, 1980) along with an increase in equivalent noise (Hawkins & Van Tasell, 1982; Thibodeau et al, 1988) and higher
total harmonic distortion (Thibodeau et al, 1988; Thibodeau & Saucedo,
1991). Therefore, each system should be evaluated on the individual user to
verify proper fit, preferably with real-ear measurements.

Headphones, Earphones.   Selection of headphones or earphones is based on
comfort, degree of hearing loss, and personal preference. Lightweight headphones offer a wide range of frequency responses and are suitable for mild to
moderate hearing losses. Feedback may be a problem with high volume-control settings. Earbuds fit in the outer ear for close coupling, providing slightly
more gain and power before feedback occurs. Dempsey and Ross (1994) reported that their subjects preferred the earbuds to headphones for comfort
and less leakage of the signal. A button receiver earphone snaps into a custom standard earmold. It increases the usable gain of a system by reducing
feedback.

Direct Audio Input.   DAI connects the receiver directly to a hearing aid. A
cord with a miniature phono plug on one end and a specialized plug consisting of two to three prongs on the other connect the device to the hearing
aid, either directly or with a boot or shoe that is slipped onto the hearing aid.
    The primary advantage of DAI is that the signal is amplified, filtered, and
processed through a hearing aid as if it had been received by the microphone. DAI allows the user to use the characteristics of his or her hearing
aid. Some hearing aids, however, change their response characteristics when
coupled to listening devices (Hawkins & Schum, 1985), so it is imperative to
ascertain how the hearing aid is responding.
    There are two primary disadvantages of DAI. The cords and connections
are fragile and tend to break easily. If the thin copper wires become twisted
or frayed, distortion may occur. Second, universal connectors for hearing
aids and listening devices do not exist. Not all hearing aids have DAI capa-
bility. The ones that are DAI compatible may not be compatible with some
auxiliary aids. The HARC Mercantile catalog (Kalamazoo, MI) devotes two
entire pages to DAI. BTEs with DAI are listed along with the corresponding
boots or shoes and cords needed to couple with devices. For example, different cords are needed when coupling to a Phonic Ear FM system (Phonic
Ear, Petaluma, CA) than when coupling to a Comtek FM system (Salt Lake
City, UT). Therefore, it is advisable to call the manufacturer of the hearing
aid and the auxiliary aid to determine if the systems are compatible and
what accessories are needed for the connection when considering DAI.

Inductive Coupling.   An alternative to the aforementioned delivery options is
the use of a telecoil, short for telephone coil. A telecoil is typically housed
within a hearing aid, although it can also be housed in a separate receiver

unit, which in turn is coupled to headphones, earbuds, or DAI. Larger hearing aids house more powerful telecoils than smaller hearing aids, thus the telecoils in body aids are more powerful than the ones in ITE aids. Does that mean that all telecoils in ITEs lack power and sensitivity? Definitely not. Telecoils can be modified to increase their strength and sensitivity by increasing the number of coils of wire or the length of the iron core; placing two telecoils in tandem, which provides an additional 6 dB; or providing a preamplifier for the telecoil. It is important to establish which manufacturers can and will make modifications in telecoils.

An important component in the use of telecoils and induction loops is the orientation of the telecoil within the hearing aid. The area of maximum pickup strength of the telecoil occurs at the ends of the metal core. Therefore, the telecoil needs to be positioned within the hearing aid to maximize its performance in any given situation. For listening devices, that position is vertical to the ground because the field generated by the induction loop is vertical. For telephone listening, the position is horizontal or diagonal to the ground. Although most manufacturers I contacted indicated that the typical placement is vertical, it would behoove all audiologists to specify the preferred direction of placement when ordering custom hearing aids or to contact the manufacturer of BTE hearing aids to ascertain the position.

The frequency response of the telecoil is also a consideration. Often audiologists and dispensers do not order telecoils because of the general belief that telecoils do not work. Research findings support that belief (Gilmore & Lederman, 1989; Rodriguez et al, 1985; Rodriguez et al, 1991) For example, Gilmore and Lederman (1989) reported that all but one of the ITEs tested in their study exhibited substantially lower gain through the telecoil than through the microphone. The typical frequency response curve from the telecoil rolled off at both low and high frequencies. The exception was an aid with a preamplifier for the telecoil. If a telecoil frequency response is not appropriate for the user's hearing loss, use of a telecoil may be more detrimental than beneficial. As more and more manufacturers include preamplifiers for telecoils and as better telecoils are built, performance through a telecoil should equal performance through a microphone.

Visual Mode

Some communication devices and many alerting devices use a visual signal to present or alert one to the presence of a sound or signal. For communication devices, the visual display of the signal may be in the form of captioning, either closed or open, offline or real-time. Closed captioning for television was introduced in 1980. In 1990, more than 400 hours of programming per week were captioned (Boone, 1990). Before enactment of the Television Decoder Circuitry Act of 1990 (Public Law 101-431), a closed-caption decoder was necessary to read the binary code transmitted on line 21 of the television signal. As of July 1, 1993, all televisions with screens 13 inches or larger were required to contain a decoder chip, which makes separate decoders unnecessary. Real-time captioning has become a popular auxiliary aid for lectures and presentations (Stuckless, 1994).

A visual signal is an effective yet silent means of alerting one to the presence of a signal. Telephones, doorbells, door knocks, smoke alarms, and alarm clocks all can be coupled to a visual display, most commonly a flashing light and most traditionally a flashing lamp. If a lamp is the signaling device, it is best to use an incandescent light bulb of 150 watts or more or a strobe light. The disadvantage of a strobe light is that it cannot be used with coded signaler, for example, one flash for the telephone, two flashes for the door.

Vibrotactile Mode

The third delivery option is through the sense of feeling. Although not limited to alerting devices, few listening devices are coupled to vibrotactile devices, although tactile aids are in common use. Alerting devices can be coupled to devices that cause a vibration or produce another sensation, such as a fan. Many people who are deaf use a fan connected to an alarm clock. Vibrators come in many sizes and shapes. Some are large and fit underneath a mattress to wake the user; some are small enough to fit under a pillow; and others may be worn on the body, either on the wrist or the waist. Delivery of a vibrotactile signal can be effective if the user is sensitive to touch and vibration and is not bothered by wearing a device.

TELECOMMUNICATIONS

The Telephone

The telephone consists of three separate subassemblies—dialing mechanism, ringer, and speech network. Connected to these is the phone line. To understand how to assist in telephone communication, a basic understanding of the telephone and factors that affect its performance is needed. The following section has been adapted from Macassey (1985).

Phone Line

The phone line is the connection between the telephone and the telephone exchange. The phone line provides the power to operate the telephone. The voltage is supplied by lead acid cells and is completely independent of the electric companies. The amount of current available, however, depends on several factors, including length of connection, impedance matching, and number of telephones in the house.

The phone line connection is usually approximately 3 miles long. If the length of the connection increases, the current available to the user decreases, a special consideration for rural users. Because the system is electrical, impedance matching is a factor. If the telephone and phone line do not have similar impedance values, a mismatch occurs. This is evidenced by an echo or whistling on the telephone line, which often occurs when inexpensive telephones are used. The third factor influencing the power available is the number of receivers off the hook. When the telephone is picked up, the line voltage drops substantially (eg, from 48 volts to 3 to 9 volts). If additional receivers are picked up, there is an even greater drop in voltage.

Dialing Mechanism

The dialing mechanism, for most household telephones, is either Touch-Tone or rotary dial. The rotary dial works by sending pulses through the lines that are produced by disconnecting the telephone at specific intervals. Touch-Tone uses audio tones.

Ringer

There are two basic types of ringers—gong ringers (the most common and the loudest) and the warble ringer. Ringers are controlled by an AC waveform that is mixed with the direct current (DC) power from the phone line. The amount of current available to drive the ringers is limited, so as ringers are added to the phone line, available current decreases. The FCC registration label on the bottom of most telephones and other devices that connect to the phone line (eg, alerting devices, answering machines) should include the ringer equivalent number (REN). This number indicates the amount of equivalent power the telephone consumes when it rings. The total REN for all the telephones and ringing devices connected to the phone lines should be less than 5B.

The total REN is an important consideration when choosing a telephone alerting device. For example, if two telephone alerting devices are needed in a situation in which three telephones are being used and if the combined total REN for the telephones is 2.2B, then devices must be selected with a combined total REN not to exceed 2.8B. Using devices that exceed this value would be more detrimental than beneficial.

Speech Network

The last component of the telephone involves the speech network. This is the component that transduces the incoming message (function of the receiver) so it can be heard and allows for the transduction of the talker's message (function of the microphone) so it can be sent to the other party. The microphone is commonly a carbon microphone, and the receiver is typically electromagnetic (Erber, 1985; Fike & Friend, 1983). In addition to sending and receiving signals, the telephone regulates the intensity of the sender's voice through the use of a side tone. Too much side tone causes speakers to lower their voices; too little side tone causes speakers to raise their voices because they perceive they cannot be heard.

Although the side tone is an invaluable feedback system, its presence can cause interference, especially in noisy environments. Most telephone microphones are not selective; any acoustic signal is picked up (some newer telephones, however, have noise-canceling microphones to assist in noisy backgrounds). If noise is present, the noise is fed back along with the speech signal through the side tone system, which causes difficulty in hearing. When the side tone is eliminated, listening improves (Holmes et al, 1983). For people with hearing impairments who frequently use the telephone in noisy situations, a mute button may be advisable. The mute button electronically disengages the microphone, eliminating the side tone. Simply placing a hand over the microphone can also improve telephone listening ability in noise (Holmes et al, 1983).

Telecommunication Options

A number of options exist to augment telecommunication (Table 6–8), including amplifying the signal through portable amplifiers, in-line amplifiers, handset amplifiers, and amplified telephones. Visual representation of the signal through computer modems, facsimiles, or text telephones (TTYs), also known as telecommunication devices for the deaf (TDDs), also is possible. The following discussion is limited to auditory enhancement devices because the visual mode of telecommunication is contraindicated for most older adults. Castle (1994) provides an in-depth discussion of visual devices.

TABLE 6–8   Telecommunication Options

PORTABLE COUPLERS
Attach to the earpiece of handset
Available as acoustic or induction devices
Offer portability and compatibility
Acoustic coupler works with all telephones
Requires battery and is not a permanent solution

HANDSET AMPLIFIERS
Replaces the original handset receiver
Compatibility depends on type of telephone and manufacturer of telephone
Considerations include style of handset, volume-control style (rotary, touchbar, amount of gain), hearing-aid compatibility, and special features (mute button, redial)

IN-LINE AMPLIFIERS
Connects between the telephone base and the handset cord
Operates similarly to handset receiver
Less expensive than handset amplifiers
More compatible than handset amplifiers

TABLE 6–8 Telecommunication Options (continued)

AMPLIFIED TELEPHONES

Replaces entire telephone

Amount of gain adjustable

Hearing-aid compatible

Most expensive option

INTERPERSONAL LISTENING DEVICES

Use of ALD with telephone

Offers advantages of ALD

Portable Couplers

If the need for portability is great, the most adaptable telephone amplifier is a portable coupler. The coupler attaches to the receiver of the handset by an elastic or detachable strap. All portable couplers operate with batteries, have volume controls, are compact enough to carry in a pocket, briefcase, or purse, and convert any telephone into a hearing-aid compatible telephone. There are two types of portable couplers: acoustic and inductive.

Although they offer a number of advantages over the other options, portable couplers are not designed to be a permanent solution. Because of the size of portable amplifiers, the telephone receiver may not be repositioned completely on the cradle with the adapter in place, necessitating removal and reattachment of the coupler each time the phone is answered or hung up. This can pose particular difficulties for older adults with poor manual dexterity. In addition, all portable adapters, whether acoustic or inductive, require batteries. If the device is left on, the batteries drain. Portable amplifiers, therefore, may be best suited for people who travel or for occasional use.

Acoustic Coupler. Acoustic couplers provide approximately 20 dB of acoustic gain (a few amplifiers provide more) and can be used on any telephone, including car telephones and cellular telephones. Because the output signal is acoustic, this coupler can be used with or without a hearing aid. In addition, acoustic couplers can be used with a telecoil because an electromagnetic field is produced during transduction of the energy. The production of the electromagnetic field also converts any telephone that is not compatible with a hearing aid into a hearing-aid compatible telephone.

Induction Coupler. An induction coupler provides slightly less gain than an acoustic coupler but is also less expensive. Because the signal is delivered solely as an electromagnetic field, use of the coupler is restricted to people who have hearing aids with telecoils. People with severe to profound hearing losses, if they have a quality telecoil, can use induction amplifiers. The coupler can be connected to accessory devices such as neckloops, plug-in silhouette inductors, or DAI systems, making the systems more flexible. For example, to maximize audibility through the use of binaural hearing aids, a neckloop or silhouette (worn on the ear opposite the induction coupler) can be coupled to the telephone coupler.

Handset Amplifiers

Amplified handsets offer a relatively inexpensive and permanent method for facilitating listening on the telephone. When the original handset is replaced with an amplified handset, output can be increased as much as 20 to 30 dB and be quite effective for most people with hearing losses.

Not all amplified handsets work with all telephones. Many amplified handsets, however, operate properly only if they are made by the same manufacturer as the telephone. Many electronic telephones, high efficiency telephones, and inexpensive telephones are not compatible. The Walker Unihandset (Walker Equipment Corp., Ringgold, GA) is, supposedly, universally compatible and designed to work on virtually any telephone. It consists of the amplified handset and a separate electronics pack that sits between the telephone and the receiver.

Selection of an amplified handset requires investigation and trial-and-error activity by audiologist and client. Even after the decision has been made that a particular handset should be compatible, there is no guarantee that it will work with the client's telephone when the telephone is connected to the phone lines in the client's house. It is advisable to allow the client to try the handset in the environment in which it is to be used. This recommendation is true for any telecommunication or alerting device.

Type of Telephone.   The first question that must be asked when considering the use of an amplified handset is the type and manufacturer of the intended telephone. The telephone must be a modular phone, that is, the handset must be detachable from the portion of the telephone that contains the dialing mechanism. Trimline and other telephones with the dialing mechanisms in the handsets are not compatible with amplified handsets. The audiologist and client must determine if the telephone is an older analog type or a new electronic type. Electronic telephones are usually the class of telephones that offer special features such as last number redial and memory. They are not compatible with a number of handsets. Clients who have not determined or cannot determine the type of telephone can be asked to describe the telephone and its features or can bring the telephone into the office with them.

Manufacturer of Telephone.   The manufacturer of the telephone must be ascertained. For many handsets, compatibility is limited to telephones made by the same manufacturer. Many patients do not know the manufacturer if the telephone is from a lesser known company. If the client does not know the name of the manufacturer, he or she can be asked the approximate cost of the telephone. Many less expensive phones are not compatible with amplified handsets because they do not provide enough power to drive the amplifiers. The same is true of high-efficiency or electronic telephones.

Style of Handset. Handsets are available in two different shapes; the mouthpiece and earpiece are either round or square. The round shape is referred to as the 500 type or G style and is the traditional handset. The square, or more modern shape, is referred to as the K style. Which style to use is primarily a personal preference, although compatibility may limit the choice.

Volume Control. There are four volume control options: rotary wheel, touchbar slide, touchbar, and three-position slide. The most common option is the rotary wheel. As the wheel is turned upward (toward the earpiece) intensity increases. As long as the wheel is unchanged, the amount of gain is unchanged. This is advantageous for people with poor manual dexterity who have difficulty manipulating the volume control with every telephone call.

The rotary wheel, however, has several disadvantages. First, the wheel is difficult to manipulate for people with poor manual dexterity. If the telephone is used by others, the person with the hearing loss constantly has to readjust the wheel to the desired level. Second, if the volume control wheel is not turned down, the volume intensity may be too great for other users of the telephone, potentially causing discomfort or damage, especially if they have normal hearing.

AT&T phones offer a touchbar slide volume control that works on the same principle as the rotary wheel. It offers the same advantages and disadvantages as rotary volume control.

The third type of volume control is the touchbar. The touchbar is operated by depressing either the top of the bar, which increases the intensity, or the bottom of the bar, which decreases the intensity. The greater the intensity desired, the more times the bar must be depressed. When the handset is replaced on the cradle, however, the amplification is disengaged. Touchbar handsets tend to be slightly more expensive than rotary dials and are less common, but they are preferable in most situations to rotary wheels. Touchbars tend to be easier to manipulate for older adults with fine-motor problems, and they safeguard the next user against overamplification.

The last, and least common, type of handset amplification is a slide bar with three volume control positions—normal, medium, and high. Because this control is discrete it does not allow minor adjustments in intensity levels. It has the same advantages and disadvantages as the rotary wheel control.

Gain. Most handsets provide approximately 20 dB of gain, under optimal situations, some providing as much as 30 dB of gain. The gain, however, may be affected by a number of variables. For example, gain may be reduced if the power from the telephone line is too low to power the amplifier or if the telephone itself lacks the necessary power to drive the handset amplifier.

Hearing-Aid Compatibility.   Most amplified handsets offer greater hearing-aid compatibility than standard receivers. That is, as the electrical signal is amplified, the strength of the electromagnetic field increases, enabling weaker and less sensitive telecoils to be more effective.

Special Features.   A number of amplified handsets offer several special features to assist a user listening in a noisy environment. One such feature is a noise-reduction or noise-canceling microphone. The other feature is the push-to-talk feature; the microphone is disengaged until the button is depressed, which activates the microphone. Both features increase the cost of the handset substantially, but the additional cost may be warranted if the listener has difficulty listening over the telephone because of the presence of background noise.

In-Line Amplifiers

In-line amplifiers are devices that are inserted between the base of the telephone and the handset. They operate on the same principle as amplified handsets but with fewer restrictions, and they offer several advantages. In-line amplifiers tend to be compatible with more telephones than are other types of amplification. Many telephones, including electronic telephones, that cannot accommodate amplified handsets operate effectively when coupled to in-line amplifiers. Because they are portable and because of their increased compatibility, in-line amplifiers are excellent devices for traveling. The initial cost of these amplifiers is lower than that of handset amplifiers, however, some require batteries that must be replaced every 6 to 12 months. The volume control is located on the device and tends to be large and easy to manipulate. Installation is simple; it is imperative, however, that the connections be made correctly. That is, the cord from the amplifier is inserted into the base of the telephone and the cord from the handset is inserted into the amplifier. The amplifier is connected between the base and the handset cord, not between the handset cord and the receiver (Figure 6–7). Many devices can be attached to the side of the telephone with two-sided tape or hook-and-loop fastener for portability. Others sit beside the telephone, although a separate device is seen as a disadvantage to many users.

Volume Control.   A rotary wheel and a sliding bar are the options for volume control. There are no distinct advantages or disadvantages between these two types of controls because the amplification does not turn off when the telephone is hung up. The choice is based on personal preference.

Gain.   Gain varies among the different in-line amplifiers, some devices offering as much as 25 dB or as little as 10 dB of gain. Again these numbers are

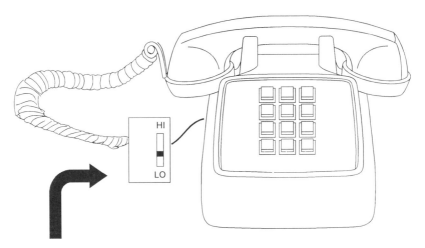

INLINE AMPLIFIER

FIGURE 6–7 *Proper connection for an in-line amplifier. The amplifier sits between the base of the telephone and the handset cord.*

reported by the manufacturers under the assumption of optimal operating conditions; therefore, the actual gain may be less.

Power Supply. In-line amplifiers are powered in one of three ways—the phone line, batteries, or a household electrical outlet. Devices that are powered by the phone line are restricted to telephones that have carbon bell ringers; newer telephones that use electronic ringers are not compatible. The choice between the other options may be dictated by the location of the telephone and the availability of electrical outlets. If there are no available outlets, devices that operate on batteries may be the only option. Devices with a low-battery indicator are preferable, when available, to indicate when new batteries are needed. The advantage of devices that require an electrical outlet is that there is no need to replace batteries. However, many of these devices are rendered useless during power outages.

Interpersonal Auxiliary Aids

Many personal listening systems can be interfaced with the telephone through a specialized connecting device. The device consists of a cord with a telephone plug, a cord with a connection to the listening device (miniature phone plug), and a telephone plug receptor. The telephone plug is inserted into the base of the telephone; the handset cord is inserted into the female receptor on the device; and the miniature phone plug is inserted into the designated jack on the listening device. The telephone signal is then routed through, and controlled by, the listening device (Figure 6–8). The user is able to listen monaurally or binaurally, with or without the use of

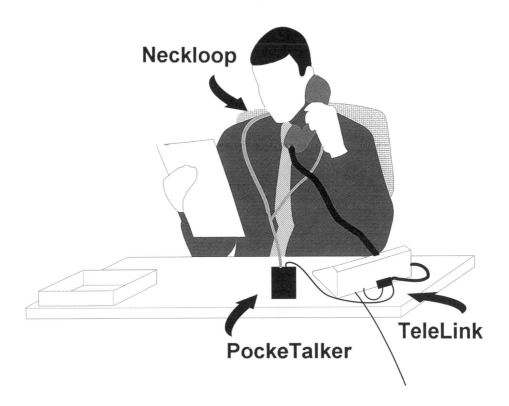

Neckloop

PockeTalker

TeleLink

FIGURE 6–8   *Use of an interpersonal listening device coupled to a telephone. The telephone handset is used only for the microphone. The telephone signal is received through the neckloop and telecoil on the hearing aids in this example.*

hearing aids, through headphones, DAI, or with a neckloop and a telecoil. The amplification of the signal is controlled through the listening device and limited only by the limits of the device. The telephone receiver is used only for the microphone.

Amplified Telephones

Amplified telephones are fully functioning telephones that offer the added feature of additional amplification. Most of these telephones are equipped with large dialing buttons and adjustable volume controls. Some have programmable memory, a lighted ringer indicator, and amplified or low-frequency audible ringers, return to normal volume when hung up, or have an additional power supply. One amplified telephone is cordless. A few have circumaural earpieces; others have traditional handsets. Some telephones are designed for mild to moderate hearing losses, offering 10 to 15 dB of gain, and others are designed for moderate to severe hearing loss with up to 40 dB of gain. One telephone can be coupled for use with a neckloop and requires fitting by a hearing care professional because it is such a powerful telephone. All amplified telephones are hearing-aid compatible.

Amplified telephones are the most expensive option presented thus far. Prices range from less than $100.00 to more than $350.00. If a client is in the market for a new telephone, however, these telephones offer an excellent means to improve telephone listening. The adjustable volume control on most telephones is easy to manipulate, especially for older adults with arthritis or reduced dexterity. With telephones that do not default to a normal volume control, there is less risk of overamplification for users with normal hearing because the volume controls are located on the base of the telephone and are easily seen. It would be prudent, however, to encourage users to return the volume control to the normal position when the telephone is hung up to eliminate any possibility of overamplification.

Alerting Devices

Historically, the older adult population with hearing impairments has not purchased alerting devices. Traditional thinking has been rather limited and may account for this lack of use.

> *Myth.* Alerting devices are flashing lamps that signal a telephone is ringing or someone is at the door.
> *Fact.* Alerting devices are any device, large or small, visual or auditory, that alerts one to the presence of a signal. An enhanced audible telephone ringer is an alerting device. Another alerting device alerts the user that the automobile blinker is still blinking, potentially averting an accident.
> *Myth.* Alerting devices are primarily for people with profound hearing losses or who are deaf. People with less severe hearing impairments are able to function with the assistance of hearing aids. Because older adults typically have mild to moderate hearing losses, they are not candidates for alerting devices.
> *Fact.* Anyone with any degree of hearing loss, regardless of age, is a candidate for an alerting device. Even while wearing amplification, many people have difficulty hearing the telephone ring, or the blinker in the car, or someone knocking on the door, especially if they are at a distance from the sound source.

It is not intended to suggest that all audiologists believe these myths. It is suggested that the audiology profession has done little to dispel them. The audiology profession has not had the foresight and knowledge to see that anyone, including older adults, with a hearing impairment of any degree may benefit from use of an alerting device. As the ADA becomes a greater driving force and audiologists become more knowledgeable about auxiliary aids, inclusion of alerting and listening devices will become routine in audiologic care.

The decision process for alerting devices follows the same steps used to choose an auxiliary device for listening. One determines how the signal will be picked up; how the signal will be transmitted; and how the signal will be delivered. The signal of an alerting device can be detected with a microphone, direct connection, or an induction connection. Transmission is usually hard-wired, but a few devices use wireless transmission. The signal can be delivered through the enhanced auditory, visual or tactile mode.

A fourth delivery mode is unique to alerting systems. For some people, the most appropriate method of signal delivery is a hearing dog. Hearing dogs are any breed of dog trained to monitor the environment of someone with a hearing impairment. The dog is trained to identify the sound source and lead the person to the source. If, for example, the doorbell is ringing, the dog leads the person to the door. When the smoke alarm is activated, however, the dog lies down on the floor rather than leading the person to the source.

Before asking the three basic questions, however, it must be decided if there is a need. For any given situation, how well the person can hear the sound or signal with and without personal amplification must be determined. Although this is an area rarely assessed in the evaluation of an older adult, it is as important as the evaluation for hearing aids. So much emphasis is placed on improving communication, audiologists fail to acknowledge that sound actually serves two other functions: background and warning (Ramsdell, 1966). How important each function is to the client plays a role in defining needs. For example, if it is important for a client's sense of safety and security to be aware of approaching footsteps, there is a great need for an alerting device. If, on the other hand, the client is not concerned and can hear with and without hearing aids a knock on the door, for example, he or she does not need an alerting device for that situation.

It is important to determine how a person performs without hearing aids. Can he or she hear the telephone? Is he or she aware of the doorbell ringing? Can he or she hear the smoke alarm in every room of the house without hearing aids and when asleep? If the answer is yes, there is little need for alerting devices. If, however, the client cannot answer yes to these questions, there is a need to investigate how alerting devices can assist the client in daily functioning. This evaluation can be easily accomplished with a listening questionnaire (Appendix 6–1). If several devices are needed, whole-house alerting systems are available. It may be more efficient to install a central system rather than several independent devices, cost permitting.

Alarm Clocks

Alarm clocks can shake, flash, or chirp loudly. Small alarms that vibrate can be tucked into a suitcase and then into a pillow to awaken one when traveling. Also available are large clocks that vibrate, flash, chirp loudly, or provide a combination of any two and can also serve as bedside lighting and indicate when the telephone is ringing. Although a few clocks are relatively expensive, others are priced the same as and are alternatives to standard alarm clocks.

Smoke Alarms

The ability to hear a smoke detector while not wearing amplification is not a luxury, it is a necessity. Although most smoke alarms emit an intense, audible signal, the alarm may not be loud enough or at a frequency that will awaken a person or to gain the attention of a person when other sounds are present. If a person finds a smoke detector difficult to hear when he or she is not wearing hearing aids, an alternative warning system must be sought.

Smoke detectors designed specifically for people with hearing impairments are available from a number of distributors. When choosing a smoke detector, the user must consider the following points: (1) Does the device meet or exceed the Underwriters Laboratories standards and the National Fire Protection Association criteria? (2) What is the most effective alarm for the user—a visual, an auditory, or vibratory signal? (3) Where will the device or devices be located? Smoke alarms must be placed strategically in the house to detect smoke as well as to warn. (4) Will the installation be portable or be permanent? To generate a signal of adequate intensity, only devices that are connected directly to the household electrical system or plug into an electrical outlet should be used. However, in power outages or if there is an electrical fire, the smoke detectors do not operate.

The ADA mandates minimum requirements for smoke detectors used in places of accommodation. Although these mandates do not apply to privately owned homes or residential dwellings, the regulations should be known and relayed to clients. Clients need to demand that every place of accommodation meets the ADA minimum for smoke detectors and warning devices, because it could be a matter of life or death.

Doorbells, Doorknocks

The ability to hear the doorbell or someone knocking on the door generates a sense of security and independence. For many older adults, this sense is compromised when they can hear the doorbell ring only if they are in the same room as the doorbell ringer. Inexpensive and easily installed devices are available to assist in these situations. The existing ringer can be replaced with a louder ringer. If that is not an option, several remote wireless doorbells are available that operate either by battery or by plugging into an electrical outlet.

For smaller living areas, such as a one-room apartment or nursing-home room, a visual display device may be more appropriate and less intrusive than an audible device. The Door Beacon (Global Assistive Devices, Inc., Ft. Lauderdale, FL), for example, can be placed on the door with hook-and-loop fastener. When someone knocks on the door, the vibration is transferred to the Door Beacon, which emits a bright flashing light.

Telephones

Devices to indicate that the telephone is ringing can be auditory or visual. Many of the devices are plugged into the telephone wall jack and are activated from the same signal that activates the telephone. Other devices attach to the telephone and detect the presence of the electromagnetic energy from the ringer and send a signal to flash a light bulb of a lamp. Others use a microphone to pick up the ringing and activate an alerting signal.

Most older adults have little difficulty hearing the telephone ring when they are in the same room as the telephone. When asked how well they hear the telephone when they are in the next room or some distance from the telephone, many have to stop to think. If there is difficulty in this situation, it may not be sufficient to increase the audibility of the telephone at the source. It may be more beneficial to provide remote devices. This is easily accomplished by using a direct-connect device plugged into the telephone jack in the other room. If no jack is present, it is possible to run a longer telephone line from an available jack to the desired room. This holds true for visual or auditory devices. When choosing devices for telephone alerting, the audiologist and client are cautioned to keep in mind that the total REN for all telephones and alerting devices should not exceed 5B.

NEEDS ASSESSMENT

For the audiologist to provide comprehensive care to a client, the audiologic evaluation must be comprehensive and thorough. The assessment cannot be limited to pure tones, speech in quiet, most comfortable loudness levels, uncomfortable loudness levels, and immittance testing. For older adults, areas of investigation should include lifestyle, living arrangements, social activities, employment, hobbies, presence of significant others, and motivation, to name a few. Other family members or significant others should be included in the evaluation. Specific to the evaluation is how well the person understands speech in everyday listening situations, on the telephone, watching television, and in an automobile and how well they are able to detect or hear environmental sounds and signals with and without the use of hearing aids.

Listening difficulties can be easily assessed with a listening questionnaire. An example of such a questionnaire is presented in Appendix 6–1.

The questionnaire can be sent to the client before the communication evaluation (a term preferred to *hearing evaluation* because it more accurately describes the intent of the evaluation) and be completed at home. The questionnaire should be reviewed during the history interview. A modified follow-up questionnaire can be sent out a few weeks or months after the communication evaluation and audiologic rehabilitation to assess the effectiveness of treatment.

Once needs have been established, the communication evaluation must proceed in finding solutions to the problems. The goal is to establish a therapeutic program to compensate for any and all aspects of the client's daily living that may be compromised by the presence of a hearing impairment. By including the assessment of listening and alerting devices in the hearing-aid evaluation, this goal is met.

CONCLUSION

Through a careful evaluation of the patient's hearing and listening needs, appropriate systems or devices can be selected to target effective communication and meet the ADA mandates. A wide variety of devices are available from a wide variety of sources. As is the case with hearing aids, selection of the devices is only the first step in the remediation process. The devices need to be incorporated into a comprehensive audiologic rehabilitation program so that the client learns how to maximize use of the device, optimize performance of the device, and minimize the effects of the hearing impairment. Appendix 6–2 presents resources pertaining to the ADA and auxiliary aids. As audiologists, the choice is ours to provide comprehensive hearing care—care that includes the use of auxiliary aids.

REFERENCES

Boone, M. (1990). This news is for you. *SHHH Journal, 11*, 29.

Castle, D.L. (1994). Telecommunications: Visual technology. In M. Ross (Ed.), *Communication access for persons with hearing loss* (pp. 145-166). Baltimore: York.

Dempsey, J.J. (1994). Hardwire personal listening systems. In M. Ross (Ed.), *Communication access for persons with hearing loss* (pp. 103-123). Baltimore: York.

Dempsey, J., & Ross, M. (1994). Evaluation of hardwired personal assistive listening devices. *American Journal of Audiology. 3*, 71-77.

Erber, N.P.(1985). *Telephone communication and hearing impairment.* San Diego: College-Hill Press.

Fike, J.L., & Friend, G.E. (1983). *Understanding telephone electronics.* Dallas: Texas Instruments.

Gilmore, R.A., & Lederman, N. (1989). Induction loop assistive listening system: Back to the future? *Hearing Instruments, 40*, 14-20.

Hawkins, D., & Schum, D. (1985). Some effects of FM-system coupling on hearing aid characteristics. *Journal of Speech and Hearing Disorders, 50*, 132-141.

Hawkins, D., & Van Tasell, D. (1982). Electroacoustic characteristics of personal FM systems. *Journal of Speech and Hearing Disorders, 47,* 355-362.

Holmes, A.E., Frank, T., & Stoker, R. (1983). Telephone listening ability in a noise background. *Ear and Hearing, 4,* 88-90.

Macassey, J. (1985). Understanding telephones. *Ham Radio, 34,* 38-44.

Palmer, C. (1992). Assistive devices in the audiology practice. *American Journal of Audiology, 1,* 37-51.

Ramsdell, D.A. (1966). The psychology of the hard-of-hearing and the deafened adult. In H. Davis & R. Silverman (Eds.), *Hearing and deafness* (pp. 459-473). New York: Holt, Rinehart & Winston.

Rodriguez, G., Holmes, A.E., & Gerhardt, K. (1985). Microphone vs telecoil performance characteristics. *Hearing Instruments, 39,* 22-24, 57.

Rodriguez, G., Meyers, C., & Holmes, A.E. (1991). Hearing aid performance under acoustic and electromagnetic coupling conditions. *Volta Review, 93,* 89-95.

Stone, R. (1993). Telecoils: Past, present, & future. *Hearing Instruments, 44,* 22-23, 26-27, 40.

Stuckless, E.R. (1994). Developments in real-time speech-to-text communication for people with impaired hearing. In M. Ross (Ed.), *Communication access for persons with hearing loss* (pp. 197-226). Baltimore: York.

Thibodeau, L. (1990). Effects of coupling FM systems to direct-input hearing aids. *Language, Speech, and Hearing Services in the Schools, 21,* 49-56.

Thibodeau, L., McCaffrey, H., & Abrahamson, J. (1988). Effects of coupling hearing aids to FM systems via neck loops. *Journal of the Academy of Rehabilitative Audiology, 21,* 49-56.

Thibodeau, L.M., & Saucedo, K.A. (1991). Consistency of electroacoustic characteristics across components of FM systems. *Journal of Speech and Hearing Research, 34,* 628-635.

Van Tasell, D., & Landin, D. (1980). Frequency response characteristics of FM miniloop auditory trainers. *Journal of Speech and Hearing Disorders, 45,* 247-258.

Veley, V.F. & Dulin, J.J. (1983). *Modern electronics: A first course.* Englewood Cliffs: Prentice Hall.

Appendix 6–1

Listening Questionnaire

Name _____ Date_____

The information you provide by completing this questionnaire will assist us in providing you with the most comprehensive service. Please circle your response for each situation. If the situation does not apply to you please circle N/A (not applicable). Thank you.

Do you now wear hearing aid(s)?   YES   NO

If your answer is NO, skip Sections I and II and complete all of sections III, IV, and V.

If your answer is YES, begin now and complete Sections I and II. For Sections I and II, answer the questions for the times you ARE wearing your hearing aid(s). Then proceed to Sections III and IV and answer for the times you ARE NOT wearing your hearing aid(s) and then complete Section V.

SECTION I. WHILE WEARING MY HEARING AID(S) I HAVE DIFFICULTY UNDERSTANDING:

In an automobile	Yes	Sometimes	No	N/A
The television	Yes	Sometimes	No	N/A
The radio	Yes	Sometimes	No	N/A
Over the telephone	Yes	Sometimes	No	N/A
In a restaurant or dining room	Yes	Sometimes	No	N/A
At a conference table	Yes	Sometimes	No	N/A
At a party	Yes	Sometimes	No	N/A
In a small family group	Yes	Sometimes	No	N/A
In the theater, movie, or play	Yes	Sometimes	No	N/A
In a house of worship	Yes	Sometimes	No	N/A
On the job	Yes	Sometimes	No	N/A

Other

(Describe on the lines below:)

_____

_____

SECTION II. WHILE WEARING MY HEARING AID(S) I HAVE DIFFICULTY HEARING

The telephone ring	Yes	Sometimes	No	N/A
When? _____				
The doorbell when I'm in another room	Yes	Sometimes	No	N/A
Someone knocking at the door	Yes	Sometimes	No	N/A
Someone calling to me from another room	Yes	Sometimes	No	N/A
When? _____				
The smoke detector at home or in hotels	Yes	Sometimes	No	N/A

If you do not wear or use hearing aid(s), start with Section III. If you do use hearing aid(s), answer the following questions for those times that you are NOT wearing your hearing aid(s).

SECTION III. WITHOUT HEARING AIDS I HAVE DIFFICULTY UNDERSTANDING

In an automobile	Yes	Sometimes	No	N/A
The television	Yes	Sometimes	No	N/A
The radio	Yes	Sometimes	No	N/A
Over the telephone	Yes	Sometimes	No	N/A
In a restaurant or dining room	Yes	Sometimes	No	N/A
At a conference table	Yes	Sometimes	No	N/A
At a party	Yes	Sometimes	No	N/A
In a small family group	Yes	Sometimes	No	N/A
In the theater, movie, or play	Yes	Sometimes	No	N/A
In a house of worship	Yes	Sometimes	No	N/A
On the job	Yes	Sometimes	No	N/A
Other				

(Describe on the lines below:)

_____

_____

SECTION IV. I HAVE DIFFICULTY HEARING

The telephone ring	Yes	Sometimes	No	N/A
When? _____				
The doorbell when I'm in another room	Yes	Sometimes	No	N/A

SECTION IV (continued). I HAVE DIFFICULTY HEARING

Someone knocking at the door	Yes	Sometimes	No	N/A
Someone calling to me from another room	Yes	Sometimes	No	N/A

When? _____

The alarm clock at home or in hotels	Yes	Sometimes	No	N/A
The smoke detector at home or in hotels	Yes	Sometimes	No	N/A

SECTION V. I HAVE KNOWLEDGE ABOUT THE FOLLOWING ITEMS

YES	NO	My rights under the Americans with Disabilities Act.
YES	NO	Devices available for alerting me to the doorbell, telephone ringing, etc.
YES	NO	Devices available to help me understand the television or radio.
YES	NO	Devices I can use on the phone to help me understand.
YES	NO	That theaters are now required to provide devices that assist me in hearing the movie or play.

That completes this questionnaire. By answering these questions you have provided a more complete picture of your listening abilities so we may be able to serve you better. Thank you again.

Appendix 6–2

Resources Pertaining to the Americans with Disabilities Act, Auxiliary Aids, and Professional Issues

1. Fanlight Productions distributes video programs about children and adults with special needs, including hearing impairments. These video tapes are available at no charge to organizations to present at conferences and for professional audiences.

Brenda Shanley
Fanlight Productions
47 Halifax Street
Boston, MA 02130
617-524-0980

2. A complete set of manuals containing step-by-step instructions on how to comply with the ADA are available from the American Speech-Language-Hearing Association (ASHA). Individual manuals or smaller sets also are available, as is a video tape.

American Speech-Language-Hearing Association
10801 Rockville Pike
Rockville, MD 20852
800-638-8255

3. Chicago has a basic resource guide for all city departments that discusses issues associated with disabilities. It is available at no charge for the first issue and then at a small fee for each additional issue.

Carol McGuire
City of Chicago Department of Personnel
City Hall, Rm 1100
121 North LaSalle St
Chicago, IL 60602
312-744-4974 (voice)
312-744-2563 (TDD)

4. Job Accommodation Network (JAN) is an organization employers can contact to receive assistance in making the place of business accessible for employees. The service is free but users are required to share their solutions with the JAN.

Job Accommodation Network
West Virginia University
809 Allen Hall
PO Box 6122
Morgantown, WV 26507-9984
800-526-7234 (voice and TDD outside WV but within the US)
800-526-4698 (voice and TDD within WV)
800-526-2262 (voice and TDD throughout Canada)

5. IBM has a National Support Center for Persons with Disabilities and provides the "Resource Guide for Persons with Hearing Impairments." It lists technology useful for persons with hearing impairments.

IBM National Support Center for Persons with Disabilities
PO Box 2150
Atlanta, GA 30301-2150
800-426-2133 (voice)
800-284-9482 (TDD)

6. Travelin' Talk is a network that offers assistance for people with disabilities who are traveling. Membership is free.

Travelin' Talk
PO Box 3534
Clarksville, TN 37043-3534
615-358-2503

7. The United States Department of Justice has an ADA hotline. The hotline is staffed by attorneys and coordinated by the Civil Rights Division.

202-514-0301 (voice)
202-514-0381 (TDD)
11:00 a.m. to 5:00 p.m. EST weekdays

8. A video tape provides instructions for using a TDD. It is a 30-minute tape that includes methods to teach others.

Sign Media, Inc.
4020 Blackburn Lane
Burtonsville, MD 20866
301-421-0268 (voice and TDD)
or
Telecommunications for the Deaf, Inc.
814 Thayer Ave
Silver Springs, MD 20910
301-589-3786 (voice and TDD)
301-589-3797 (fax)

9. Guidelines for new construction and alterations for meeting ADA mandates are available at no cost.

Architectural Transportation Barriers Compliance Board
1331 F St, NW
Suite 1000
Washington, DC 20004-1111

202-272-5434 (voice and TDD)

202-272-5447 (fax)

10. Video tapes and reference information are available from Self Help for Hard of Hearing People (SHHH). Publications concern communication access, the ADA, consumer rights, hearing loss, and other topics. Minimal fee.

SHHH Publications

7910 Woodmont Ave.

Suite 1200

Bethesda, MD 20814

301-657-2248 (voice)

301-657-2249 (TDD)

11. A list of classic Hollywood films and video cassettes that are captioned is updated every 6 months.

Anna S. Hall

Caption Club, NCI

5203 Leesburg Pike

Falls Church, VA 22041

703-998-2400 (voice and TDD)

12. Text Telephone Directories are available for a fee.

Telecommunications for the Deaf, Inc.

8719 Colesville Rd, Suite 300

Silver Springs, MD 20910

301-589-3766 (voice)

301-589-3006 (TDD)

13. The following organizations have brochures that discuss various aspects of hearing loss, ADA, and auxiliary aids. Contact them for copies and ordering instructions.

Consumer Affairs Division

ASHA

10801 Rockville Pike

Rockville, MD 20852

800-638-8255

The Canadian Hearing Society

Head Office

271 Spadina Rd

Toronto, Ontario, Canada M5R 2V3

416-964-9595 (voice)

416-964-0023 (TDD)

SHHH

7910 Woodmont Ave

Suite 1200

Bethesda, MD 20814

301-657-2248 (voice)

301-657-2249 (TDD)

14. The following books or references are appropriate for an audiologist's professional library.

ADA Handbook
Equal Employment Opportunity Commission
1801 L St, NW
Washington, DC 20507
800-669-3362 (voice)
800-669-3302 (TDD)
American Journal of Audiology Palmer, C. (1992). Assistive devices in audiology practice. *1*, 37-51. Excellent bibliography.
Assistive Devices: Doorways to Independence
Book and videotape by C. Compton and Gallaudet University
Academy of Dispensing Audiologists
3008 Millwood Ave.
Columbia, SC 29205
800-445-8629
How to Comply with The Americans with Disabilities Act: A Detailed Guide
Business & Legal Reports, Inc.
39 Academy St.
Madison, CT 06443-1513
800-727-5257 (voice)
203-245-2559 (fax)
Legal Rights: The Guide for Deaf and Hard-of Hearing People DuBow, S., Geer, S., & Peltz Strauss, K. (1992). Washington: Gallaudet University Press
800 Florida Ave. NE
Washington, DC 20002
202-651-5373
15. The following is a list of resources:
Civil Rights Division
Office of the Americans with Disabilities Act
Department of Justice
PO Box 66118
Washington, DC 20035-6118
National Center for Law and Deafness
Gallaudet University
800 Florida Ave, NE
Washington, DC 20002-3695
202-651-5373 (voice and TDD)
National Institute on Disabilities and Rehabilitation Research
US Department of Education
400 Maryland Ave, SW
Washington, DC 20202-25725
202-732-1134 (voice)
202-732-5079 (TDD)

Underwriters Laboratories, Inc.
Publications Stock
333 Pfingsten Rd
Northbrook, IL 60062
708-272-8800

Chapter 7

Older Adults in Long-Term Care Facilities

Diane Shultz and Richmond B. Mowry

As pointed out in Chapter 1, only a small proportion of older adults reside in long-term care facilities. However, because of the high prevalence of hearing loss in this population, the unique problems and needs of the elderly who live in institutions must be realized. They are addressed in this chapter. Voeks et al (1990) found that only 24 percent of residents of nursing homes they assessed could be classified as having hearing within normal limits. Schow and Nerbonne (1980) found that 70 to 80 percent of residents of nursing homes have hearing losses. Half of these patients have severe losses.

The American Speech-Language-Hearing Association (ASHA) (1988) outlined a number of resident care services that audiologists can provide. In addition to the identification, evaluation, and rehabilitation of residents with hearing losses, ASHA suggested that important areas of focus for older adults in institutions include hearing-aid orientation, counseling, environmental manipulation training, and auditory and visual speech recognition training.

An audiologist who provides services within long-term care facilities has an important role in evaluating the relative contributions of hearing impairment and cognitive decline to the confusion, disorientation, and depression frequently observed in residents of nursing homes. Weinstein and Amsel (1986) reported that 70 percent of elderly patients in institutions who were not demented and 83 percent of elderly patients in institutions who were demented were hearing impaired. They showed that hearing loss can present symptoms similar to those of dementia. When a patient in an institution responds inappropriately to a question, it might be due to hearing loss, dementia, or a combination of the two. Weinstein and Amsel (1986), for example, compared patients' performance on the Short Portable Mental Status Questionnaire (Pfeiffer, 1975) with and without use of an auditory trainer. Nearly half of patients with moderate hearing losses and all of the patients with severe losses had clinically significant improvements in their cognitive test results when tests questions were amplified. Some patients did not show significant improvements in their overall mental status scores, but the answers they gave, although wrong, were more appropriate for the types of questions asked.

In a study of 263 patients in a nursing home, Witte (1989) investigated the relation between patient age, cognitive status, degree of hearing loss, speech discrimination, and receptivity to use of a hearing aid. The results indicated that the characteristic that appeared to have the greatest impact on audiologic rehabilitation was the patient's cognitive status. The patients with cognitive impairments, regardless of age, were more likely to reject hearing-aid fittings, even after a trial period. Witte (1989) offered several suggestions for increasing acceptance of hearing aids among patients with cognitive impairments who live in institutions. In Witte's experience, care in hearing-aid fittings (eg, fitting patients with postauricular hearing aids with tamper-resistant battery compartments) and guidance of caregivers resulted in greater likelihood that patients, even those with Alzheimer disease, would benefit from and use hearing aids.

The effect of hearing loss on residents of extended-care facilities was described by Griffin et al (1988). According to these authors, hearing loss can exacerbate other functional limitations, leading to depression, isolation, stress, and frustration. Audiologists can play a pivotal role in improving the quality of life for residents of nursing homes.

Over the years, audiologists and speech-language pathologists have given increased attention to the provision of hearing care and in-service training in extended-care facilities. As Kricos and Gipson (1981) showed, it is imperative that communication specialists be sensitive to the characteristics and needs of personnel and residents of nursing homes. Effective in-service training and patient care can be planned and implemented if the professional is aware of the unique characteristics of the nursing-home environment.

Audiologists who work in long-term care facilities are particularly challenged to provide effective and appropriate services to residents with dementia, especially those with Alzheimer disease. Alzheimer disease occurs in approximately half of cases of dementia, and at this time cannot be reliably diagnosed except at autopsy. There is no effective treatment to reverse or delay the effects of the disease, although medical researchers continue to investigate the disease process (Kistner, 1993).

Voelkl (1993) showed that the difficulties of planning appropriate interventions for residents with dementia are compounded by the high prevalence of depression among older adults with dementia. Voelkl emphasized the need to consider interventions that will enhance residents' perceptions of control and well-being. Although Voelkl (1993) did not mention hearing impairment specifically, it seems plausible that reduction of hearing handicap through amplification and audiologic rehabilitation might be an important means of helping residents with depression and hearing losses gain a higher degree of self-perceived control and well-being. Neidhart and Allen (1993) emphasized the importance of involving families of the elderly in planning interventions. They wrote that clinicians must meet with all members of the family to assess needs, resources, and problems. Involving the families of residents with dementia in the selection of hearing aids and other interventions should enhance the likelihood of success of audiologic rehabilitation.

There is a need for hearing health care in long-term care facilities, but the road to providing this care is fraught with many difficulties and obstacles. Bloom (1994) described a number of the challenges and rewards of providing hearing care in long-term care facilities. The emphasis in the remainder of this chapter is a workable, practical approach to providing hearing care within nursing homes. Six problem areas are delineated as being frequently encountered by audiologists and speech-language pathologists who serve long-term care facilities. Each of these areas is discussed by Diane Shultz and Richmond B. Mowry, audiologists who provide services to long-term care facilities in Arizona and Colorado, respectively. At the end of the chapter, Shultz describes her approach to in-service training and service provision, and Mowry describes a full-service audiology program for patients in a nursing home.

PROBLEMS IN SERVING A LONG-TERM CARE CENTER

Visiting the Center and Finding the Patient

Shultz

Anyone who has visited a nursing home to care for a patient realizes that visits can turn into time-consuming and frustrating experiences. One common hurdle is finding the patient. The staff often has no idea where the patient may be, and there are a number of places in a center where a resident can temporarily disappear. Appropriate places to check include the bathroom, dining hall, and the activity room.

Sometimes finding the patient is no guarantee that a service visit will be accomplished promptly. If the patient is playing bingo or engaged in a sing-along, it may be difficult to get him or her back to the room for a test or check of the hearing aid.

> On one unforgettable occasion, my patient was in the bathroom when I arrived. She called out to me to come in and help her, believing I was the nurse. I responded that I was the audiologist and rang for help. As my patient continued to yell loudly and with no immediate relief in sight, I went to her rescue. While I was helping her, my patient berated me for taking so long and for not knowing what I was doing (which was true). As I escorted her back to her bed, the patient suddenly looked at me and said, "Diane, what are you doing here?" I explained that I was there to check and clean her hearing aids and proceeded to do just that.

Poorly planned nursing home visits do not benefit either the audiologist or the patient. The audiologist should have a scheduled appointment to see the patient (not at mealtimes) and call the day of the appointment to make sure the patient is there and feeling well enough to be seen. This simple precaution will prevent many frustrating experiences.

Mowry

Patients are residents. The facility is their home, and the residents have specific routines they follow each day as well as specific routines set by the facility. Professionals should respect the patient's home as they would any other home they visit. One should knock on the door before entering the room and greet the resident.

The appointment should be for a specific day and time and should not interfere with an activity that is important to the patient. When making the appointment, the audiologist should speak with the resident first. If the patient has dementia, the appointment should be scheduled through the social worker. People to notify when scheduling an appointment are the patient, the family, the nursing staff, and the social worker. All are important in administrative policy.

If the appointment is for a hearing evaluation, the audiologist must first have a written doctor's order—preferably a telephone order that is kept in the patient's medical chart. It is extremely important that the audiologist keep a copy for his or her records. If Medicare and Medicaid are being billed, specific wording is required on the doctor's order.

The best times for appointments are 6:30 a.m. (before breakfast); 9:30 a.m. (after breakfast); and 1:30 p.m. (after lunch). Other times usually interfere with activities or visits by family. In some situations it is important to have family present for the hearing evaluation or hearing-aid fitting.

Cerumen Management

Shultz

Cerumen management practices vary from facility to facility. The best care centers, when advised of impacted wax, order use of a softening agent for 5 days followed by ear lavage. Audiologists who have a good working relationship with the staff usually find that their lavage recommendations are carried out. Often, however, the nursing staff cannot proceed without a physician's order. If the audiologist and the physician have a good rapport, the physician will act on the audiologist's advice. The worst situation for audiologists is finding it difficult, if not impossible, to have the order issued or to find that an issued order has not been carried out. This happens more often than it should. The solution requires education for the nursing staff and physicians. Now that it is within the scope of practice for appropriately trained audiologists to perform cerumen management, some of these problems can be eliminated.

Mowry

Otoscopy is a critical procedure when seeing a resident of a nursing home. In more than 60 nursing homes I screened, an average of 30 percent of residents required cerumen management after initial otoscopy. Of these, 50 percent required routine cerumen management either monthly or quarterly. It is surprising that most nursing homes have no otoscope. When an otoscope is present, few nurses know proper otoscopy techniques or the anatomy of the ear. Cerumen management is often performed only when the problem is detected—usually by an audiologist. In-service training and patience are appreciated by the administrator, director of nursing, and nursing staff. The most appreciative person is the patient. Now that cerumen management falls within their scope of practice, audiologists must become experts in this area and provide this service to patients. Some patients, however, require the attention of an otorhinolaryngologist when impaction is severe.

Lost Hearing Aids

Shultz

Lost hearing aids are an important problem for all concerned. Most facilities do the best they can to prevent hearing aids from getting lost, but misplaced hearing aids are a common occurrence. Often the patient puts the hearing aid in a pocket and the aids ends up in the laundry.

A number of the care centers have the night nurse place the patient's hearing aid in a plastic bag labeled with the patient's room and bed number. The next morning the day nurse returns the aid and makes sure the patient wears it. Patients who are alert enough to insert their own hearing aids usually keep the aids and the batteries in a drawer by the bed.

> I have a patient in a nursing home that I visit each month for service. On one occasion the nurse at the facility had called and said that Mr. G's ear was sore and needed to be checked. On arrival, I discovered that Mr. G had a sore ear because he was wearing someone else's earmold and hearing aid. When I called this to the attention of the staff, the nurse proceeded to open a drawer that contained approximately a dozen hearing aids and said, "Take a look in there and see if his is one of those." This was not the first time I looked for a patient's hearing aid in a drawer, and it probably will not be the last. Taking care of small hearing aids received low priority from the overworked and underpaid staff.

Mowry

Hearing aids are lost in nursing homes at an alarming rate. Control of hearing aids is greatly increased when patients are categorized by their ability to physically and mentally care for their own hearing aid. If the patient has difficulty, direct control of the hearing aid should become the responsibility of the nursing staff. The hearing aid is fitted to the patient in the morning or during specified times and then retrieved in the evening.

Finding a lost hearing aid is easier when a safety cord is attached. I use color-coded cords for my patients (red for the right ear and blue for the left ear). The cord is permanently attached to the hearing-aid case with a screw or safety loop. A clothing clip is attached to the other end, and a small name tag is placed on the cord. Use of the cord system has reduced the loss factor at my nursing homes by over 80 percent. All the hearing aids in the nursing home are identified by manufacturer and serial number and kept on record with the social worker. This system works well to identify hearing aids that are found without name tags. This has become a popular and much-needed service for patients in nursing homes.

Physician and Staff Involvement

Shultz

One of the greatest obstacles that prevents audiologists from providing quality hearing services in care centers is that the physicians and staff have important health issues to deal with and often do not consider hearing loss to be significant. Although communication is important to the overall mental health of a person, many patients in a nursing home have serious illnesses that consume the attention of the medical staff. The day-to-day tasks of providing personal care such as bathing, shaving, and dressing take time. It is a time-consuming responsibility to prepare patients for meals and feed them. Many patients with dementia are demanding and difficult to care for. It is understandable, therefore, that staff often view hearing loss and hearing aids as just one more time-consuming task on a list of a great many. As a result, physicians and staff often do not attach the same importance to improving the hearing of residents of nursing homes that audiologists do. Some physicians, in fact, wrongly assume that hearing aids are inappropriate for patients with dementia. The following personal experiences illustrate this statement.

> My colleagues and I were asked to visit a care facility to evaluate a patient's hearing and make appropriate recommendations regarding amplification for a woman whose condition was diagnosed as senile dementia. The patient was aggressive and difficult for the nursing staff to care for. After testing, I recommended that the patient be given a 30-day trial period with amplification in one ear to determine if better hearing would help her become responsive and easier for the staff to care for. The patient's son, who had requested the evaluation, signed a medical waiver. The aid was fit and the patient's progress was monitored by me and the staff of the nursing home. Both the nursing staff and the social worker at the care center reported that the patient was more responsive and communication with her was easier. The physician, however, refused to sign the medical clearance form I had sent him with a

copy of the patient's audiogram and a full report. He stated that the patient's problem was not hearing loss but dementia and that he would not recommend a hearing aid. The son asked us to take back the hearing aid because the doctor did not give "permission" for his mother to have it.

A similar incident with a happier ending involved a man whose condition was diagnosed as Alzheimer disease and who had a history of several cerebrovascular accidents. The wife of the patient signed the medical waiver because she noticed how much more responsive her husband was when he was wearing the hearing aid. This patient is still wearing his aid and his wife is pleased with the results of amplification.

In each situation a physician had been contacted both by letter and in person so the audiologist could explain the audiologic results and emphasize that these patients had responded favorably to amplification. Educating physicians to the importance of hearing and the benefits of amplification should be an overriding concern for audiologists. Unfortunately, however, many audiologists in private practice either work alone or have a small staff and lack the time required to implement a comprehensive educational program.

I send monthly mailings to more than 200 physicians in my community. I use colored postcards titled *Audiology Tip of the Month*, which contain educational information. Topics include "Communicating with the Hearing Impaired," "The Americans with Disabilities Act," "How to Interpret the Audiogram," "Wax Management for Those Who Wear Hearing Aids," "Psychologic Effects of Hearing Loss," and "Hearing Aids: Monaural Versus Binaural." I have had positive comments from the medical community regarding these mailings. Physicians are busy, and the postcard format ensures that the message is brief and to the point. Too often audiologists are overwhelmed with the task of educating others about hearing loss, but we can each reach out to our own community and teach those in our immediate vicinity. If the profession as a whole takes the responsibility, the impact can be tremendous. Too often we have left the responsibility for education to others with the result that physicians and the community do not look to us for expertise in hearing care. Audiologists should be the first professionals the public and other professions turn to for answers regarding hearing problems.

Mowry

When I believe a patient may be helped with a hearing evaluation or hearing aid, I make it a point to discuss my impression with the family, social worker, nursing staff, and the attending physician. My impressions and recommendations usually are accepted. For patients with dementia I always emphasize to all concerned that this is a trial fitting and that the final decision is made during a rehabilitation staff meeting. If there is no improvement in the patient's communication ability, the hearing aid is returned.

It is the nurses' responsibility to care for a patient's hearing aid if the patient is unable to do so. In some situations nursing assistants and other ancillary staff members perform this duty. Considering the high turnover of these personnel, there is not enough time to train them each month. Nurses are usually stable in their employment and are most appropriate for this type of care. Audiologists who find that nurses are not performing hearing-aid care should ask the director of nursing to distribute a policy statement on the responsibility for hearing-aid care.

Personnel Turnover

Shultz

An issue of concern in providing care in nursing homes is the high turnover of personnel in these facilities. When it seems that all nurses and nursing assistants have been trained, they leave, and a whole new staff has to be educated. Audiologists must be willing to offer in-service training on a regular basis to ensure that all staff receive exposure to the program. The residents deserve the best possible care regarding their hearing loss and care of their hearing aids, and only an adequately educated staff can provide this care on a day-to-day basis.

Mowry

Annual in-service training for all nurses and ancillary staff is critical for the success of any nursing-home audiology program. It is important to offer continuing education credits. A trouble-shooting guide on hearing aids should be provided at each nurse's station. While in the nursing home, the audiologist should provide brief, on the spot, in-service training to all staff members when applicable. The audiologist should provide a hearing health care policy statement to be added to the rules and regulations of the facility. This policy requires all staff to be educated in the proper care of residents of nursing homes who are hard of hearing.

Family Involvement and Reimbursement Issues

Shultz

It is important that the patient's family be involved in any decision-making regarding amplification. A state such as Arizona that caters to winter visitors has the additional challenge of trying to contact families who may live in another state. Long-distance phone calls are time-consuming and expensive, but communication with the nearest relative or the decision-making family member is imperative if the hearing needs of the patient are to be met.

Arizona does not have a Medicaid program that pays for hearing aids for adults on a routine basis. The only time a program pays for hearing aids for adults is when the aid can be proved to be a medical necessity. A program called the Community Hearing Aid Program (CHAP) addresses the needs of those who cannot afford hearing aids. In this program, a network of hearing care professionals donate their time for the hearing-aid fittings and charge only a minimal amount for the actual hearing aids for those who otherwise could not obtain hearing aids because of lack of finances. There is a long waiting period (approximately 1 year), and the service covers only a small percentage of those needing amplification. The Lions Club also has a hearing aid program for the needy, but children are first on the list. When there is a surplus of hearing aids, adults are fitted.

Mowry

It is important to involve the family when trying to make a decision regarding amplification. Before the initial audiologic evaluation, the family always must be contacted for information on the patient's hearing and amplification history. Quite often, appropriate amplification devices have been purchased and are being kept by a family member. Some family members are reluctant to release the hearing aid to the nursing home for fear that it will be lost. The audiologist should explain the safety-cord program for amplification devices and see that such a program exists at the patient's facility. Assuring family members that the nursing staff has been trained to care for the hearing aid often puts the hearing aid where it is supposed to be—on the patient.

When fitting a new amplification device to a patient, I make it mandatory that the speech-language pathologist be present, because in most facilities, it is the speech-language pathologist who provides auditory rehabilitation and communication therapy. I also encourage the speech-language pathologist to involve family members in at least two of the auditory rehabilitation therapy sessions.

Regarding reimbursement issues, there are two types of patients in the nursing home setting—the private-pay patient who pays for the device "out of pocket," and the Medicaid patient who has no funds for such a purchase. The private-pay patient is regarded as any patient who visits a private clinic. The Medicaid patient is one who does not have the use of their income other than a small amount for personal needs each month. Most of Medicaid patients' monthly income is used for the expense of receiving nursing home care. Typically each state has its own Medicaid program for the purchase of amplification devices. Because state laws differ, it is important for audiologists to know the rules and regulations in their particular locales.

Colorado uses a little known federal law to assure that Medicaid patients receive medical and remedial care that is not subject to payment by Colorado Medicaid or third-party insurance. The process of making all allowable reductions in a patient's income before calculating the patient's payment to a nursing facility is called *posteligibility treatment of income* (PETI). The list of allowable reductions was expanded considerably by the Medicare Catastrophic Coverage Act of 1988. As of April 8, 1988, clients in institutions may deduct certain medical expenses from their income before obligation of patient payment is calculated. These deductions must be for incurred expenses for medical or remedial care that are not subject to payment by Colorado Medicaid or third-party insurance. These expenses include health insurance premiums, deductibles, or coinsurance; dental care; hearing aids, supplies, and care; corrective lenses, eye care, and supplies; and other incurred expenses for medical or remedial care that are not subject to payment by a third party.

The program in Colorado has worked well for Medicaid patients with hearing impairments. The audiologist is usually paid 1 to 2 months after the expense is approved; the approval process can take 1 to 2 months.

PROVIDING IN-SERVICE TRAINING TO NURSING HOME STAFF (SHULTZ)

It is necessary to contact the director of nursing to schedule an in-service training session at a time that is convenient for the staff. I offer to provide in-service training sessions for each shift because all staff members should be educated in hearing health care. The second and third shifts are often neglected when it comes to training.

Topics covered during an in-service should include a brief description of the anatomy of the ear, communication problems of people with hearing impairments, tips for communicating with patients who are hard-of-hearing, tinnitus, how to check and change a battery (I leave a battery tester with the director of nursing), and how to trouble-shoot hearing aids. Trouble-shooting topics should include checking for wax in earmolds or receivers and making sure the hearing aid is not turned off or in the T position. The staff should be shown how to check to make sure the hearing aid or earmold fits properly. Nurses and assistants need to be taught what feedback is and how to check for possible causes. I provide a number of different styles of hearing aids and earmolds so that participants receive hands-on experience.

In-service training provides a good opportunity to discuss ways of keeping track of hearing aids. I recommend that the patient's hearing aid be listed in the chart on the inventory list. The name, model, serial number, battery size, and the ear the aid fits (if monaural) should be recorded. Nancy McBride, a speech-language pathologist with Phoenix-based Nova Care, has instituted a good tracking system in her care centers. She posts a trouble-shooting guide at the nurses' station with a list of the room and bed numbers of patients who wear hearing aids. Copies of the trouble-shooting guide on red paper are posted above the bed of each patient as a reminder to the staff (Appendix 7–1). I suggest that the name and serial number of the hearing aids, battery size, and which ear the hearing aid fits be written on the master list. This plan does not take much time or effort and would reduce the number of misplaced or lost hearing aids. Formal in-service training sessions should be conducted each year, and ongoing informal training should take place every time the audiologist is in the facility.

SETTING UP A SERVICE PROGRAM (SHULTZ)

The type of program an audiologist establishes depends on the number of staff members available to oversee the program. One way to implement a hearing program in a nursing home is to contact the administrator and offer to screen all the residents in the facility at no charge in exchange for exclusive hearing-aid referrals. When all patients have undergone screening, a schedule can be set up for the audiologist to visit the facility once a month to screen all new patients.

The initial hearing screening begins with an otoscopic examination to rule out impacted cerumen and to assess the integrity of the tympanic membrane. If there is impacted wax, verbal and written orders are given to the nursing staff to have the wax removed. Patients who pass the otoscopic examination are screened with pure-tone tests. If the patient can walk or can be moved, testing should be conducted in a quiet room. Most facilities are cooperative in finding a suitable area for testing. If the patient must stay in bed, hearing can be screened with a Welch Allyn AudioScope (Welch Allen, Inc., Skaneateles Falls, NY) at bedside. When hearing is screened with an audiometer, a 30 decibel hearing level (dB HL) tone is used at 1000 Hz, 2000 Hz, and 4000 Hz. When the environment is quiet enough, 500 Hz may be tested. When a patient does not respond appropriately to a pure-tone screening, an oral hearing screening is used. A sample screening is included in Appendix 7–2.

Patients who do not pass the otoscopic screening are rescheduled for a pure-tone screening when the ears are clear. Those who do not pass pure-tone or oral hearing screening are scheduled for a complete hearing evaluation pending medical referral. The medical referral is essential if the audiologist is to be reimbursed for the testing.

The diagnostic evaluation should include the following steps:

1. Audiologic case history (Appendix 7–3)
2. Otoscopic examination to assess the integrity of the external canal and tympanic membrane
3. Pure-tone threshold tests (air and bone) with appropriate masking. The pure-tone tests are used to determine the type and severity of the hearing loss.
4. Speech recognition threshold and word recognition tests to determine the patient's ability to detect, discriminate, and understand speech
5. Immittance audiometry to determine middle ear function

It is often necessary to modify the formal test battery when the patient is not able to respond by raising a hand or finger. Some of the same techniques used for testing children may be used for these patients. I perform speech testing first to assess the hearing level and have the patient point to body parts or spondee pictures to obtain the speech recognition threshold. I also use pictures when testing word recognition. A simplified word recognition test requires the patient to identify familiar pictures or objects in the room. One patient, who could not respond appropriately to the W-22 word list, was able to repeat the names of states and answer questions about his past occupation. I often have the patients clap, nod their head, or say "yes" when they hear the tone. It is easier for patients to respond to pulsed tones rather than a steady tone.

I report the test results orally to the nurse on duty, director of nursing, social activities director, and speech-language pathologist. The test information is also recorded in the patient's chart along with any audiologic rehabilitation recommendations. A copy of the audiogram is put in the chart, and a complete report is sent to the patient's physician along with recommendations. I contact the closest family member (listed in the chart) and let him or her know the outcome of the testing both orally and with a written report. If amplification is indicated, I inform the family that the patient will have a 30-day trial period with the hearing aid and that the patient's progress will be checked weekly. I assure them that it will be the combined recommendations of staff and family that will determine whether or not the patient keeps the hearing aids.

I often fit hearing aids with a screw-set volume control and include some type of compression to help control the loud noises the patient encounters in a nursing home. A health care professional who sells a hearing aid to a patient in a long-term care facility must ensure that the patient is able to adjust the amplification, that the patient receives support from staff and family, and that the hearing aid makes a difference in the patient's ability to communicate. When the decision is made to purchase the hearing aid, a follow-up program must be instituted to make sure the patient continues to use the amplification. The staff needs to be reminded to check the batteries and to call the audiologist when there is a problem. I schedule visits twice a year for preventive maintenance. At these visits I check the patient's ear for wax, clean and check the hearing aid, and make sure the patient is wearing the hearing aid. Once a year the patient's hearing is re-evaluated.

A SUCCESSFUL AUDIOLOGY SERVICE PROGRAM
FOR PATIENTS IN A NURSING HOME (MOWRY)

No group of older adults has more special needs than adults with hearing impairments who live in nursing homes. Appendix 7– 4 is an outline of a successful full-service program for patients in nursing homes who are hard-of-hearing and who are at a disadvantage in communication. The more audiologists share ideas in areas that demand and challenge clinical expertise, the more they will develop creative knowledge through failures and successes. Audiology will become a better profession when individual practitioners care for patients who traditionally have been ignored.

My background in nursing-home care for adults with hearing impairments included a position with a national rehabilitation corporation that specializes in nursing-home rehabilitation of patients who require physical therapy, occupational therapy, speech therapy, or audiologic service. I also own a private practice in which 90 percent of the patients are residents of nursing homes.

I agree with Shultz that few audiologists are enthusiastic about seeing patients who live in nursing homes. Those who are not familiar with the nursing-home environment usually find themselves surrounded by unpleasant sights and smells, which usually means a quick visit and a return to a peaceful, quiet, environmentally controlled office. Nursing homes have been preyed upon for years by unethical practitioners who seek a quick sale only to leave the patient with a hearing aid but no auditory rehabilitation or communication therapy or regular care. This growing population is in great need of professional services. They have been ignored by our profession for far too long.

REFERENCES

American Speech-Language-Hearing Association (1988). Provision of audiology and speech-language pathology services to older persons in nursing homes. *ASHA, 30*, 72-74.

Bloom, S. (1994). Hearing care in nursing homes offers daunting challenges, special rewards. *Hearing Journal, 47*, 13-20.

Griffin, K., Tourigny, A., & Demitrack, L. (1988). The hearing-impaired population in U.S. nursing homes. *Hearing Instruments, 39*, 6-8.

Kistner, M.A. (1993). Alzheimer's disease. In T.O. Blank (Ed.), *Topics in gerontology: Selected annotated bibliographies* (pp. 141-155). Westport: Greenwood.

Kricos, P., & Gipson, G. (1981). A bilateral approach to awareness raising in skilled nursing facilities. *Communicative Disorders, 6.*

Neidhart, E.R., & Allen, J.A. (1993). *Family therapy with the elderly.* Newbury Park: SAGE.

Pfeiffer, E. (1975). A short portable mental status questionnaire for the assessment of organic brain deficit in elderly patients. *Journal of the American Geriatrics Society, 10*, 433-441.

Schow, R., & Nerbonne, M. (1980). Hearing levels among elderly nursing home residents. *Journal of Speech and Hearing Disorders, 45*, 124-132.

Voeks, S., Gallagher, C., Langer, E., & Drinka, P. (1990). Hearing loss in the nursing home: An institutional issue. *Journal of the American Geriatrics Society, 38*, 141-145.

Voelkl, J.E. (1993). Activity among older adults in institutional settings. In J.R. Kelly (Ed.), *Activity and aging: Staying involved in later life* (pp. 231-246). Newbury Park: SAGE.

Weinstein, B., & Amsel, L. (1986). Hearing loss and dementia in the institutionalized elderly. *Clinical Gerontologist, 4*, 3-15.

Witte, K. (1989). Hearing impairment and cognitive decline among aging nursing home patients. *Hearing Journal, 42*, 17-20.

Appendix 7–1

How to Pinpoint Problems with Your Hearing Aid (Diane Schultz)

The following checklist offers general guidelines for trouble-shooting problems with hearing aids.

- If the hearing aid does not work, replace the battery with a new one.
- Is the battery in backward?
- Is the sound intermittent? Contact the audiologist.
- Is there wax in the opening at the end of the canal? If so, clean it with an old toothbrush or wax loop.
- Is the battery compartment closed tightly?
- Is the volume turned up?
- Is there corrosion on the battery? If so, rub the battery ends with a rough cloth or a rubber pencil eraser.
- Does a whistling sound occur while the aid is in the ear? A certain amount of feedback may result when a hand or other solid object is placed near the ear. This is not necessarily abnormal; however, no feedback should occur at other times. Inappropriate feedback may result from wax impaction, a loosely fitting hearing aid or earmold, or incomplete insertion. Consult the audiologist if there is trouble with feedback.
- Is the amplification intermittent or does crackling occur when you manipulate the volume control? If so, consult the audiologist.

Appendix 7–2

Hearing Screening Form (Diane Shultz)

Facility _____   Date of Admission _____
Patient _____   Date of Screening _____

1. The patient should answer the following questions when asked by examiner with normal loudness and no repetition.

How are you? _____

What is your name? _____

What did you have for breakfast, lunch, dinner? _____

Where were you born? _____

Do you have any family? _____What are their names? _____

When is your birthday? _____

2. Localization
Was the patient able to determine where you were and what was said?

_____

3. Identification
Was the patient able to repeat:

bass/band/bath	_____	_____	_____
zoo/shoe/Sue	_____	_____	_____
come/bum/gum	_____	_____	_____
two/due/new	_____	_____	_____
that/they/them	_____	_____	_____
man/pat/bad	_____	_____	_____

4. Subjective observations (need for repetition, inaccurate responses, speechreading skills, etc):

_____

_____

5. Recommendations

Hearing evaluation _____

Rescreen _____

No recommendation _____

Appendix 7–3

Audiologic Case History (Diane Shultz)

Name _____   Date of Birth _____
Facility _____   Audiologist _____

BACKGROUND INFORMATION

Have you had your hearing tested before? _____   When? _____
When did you first notice you had a hearing problem? _____
Which do you think is the better hearing ear? _____
Which ear do you use when talking on the phone? _____
Did your hearing become worse all of a sudden or was the loss gradual?
_____
Do you have good and bad days with your hearing? _____
Does it fluctuate? _____
Do you have any buzzing or ringing in your ears? _____
Are you ever dizzy? Describe: _____
Do loud sounds bother you? _____
Have you ever worked in or been exposed to loud noises? _____
Does anyone on your side of the family have a hearing problem? _____
Do you have any pain or drainage from the ears? _____
Have you ever had any ear surgery? _____
Family physician: _____
Address: _____

COMMUNICATION PROBLEMS

Where do you have trouble hearing? Radio or television _____
Groups _____ One on one _____
Do you hear but have difficulty in understanding? _____
Do you avoid social situations because of your hearing problem? _____
Do you hear and understand men better than women or children? _____

AMPLIFICATION HISTORY

Have you ever worn a hearing aid? _____ If yes, please answer the following:
Type(s): _____
Ear(s) fitted: _____ Brand(s): _____
When purchased: _____
Do you have any physical limitations that make it difficult to manipulate
small controls? _____

Appendix 7–4

Full-Service Audiology Program for Residents of a Nursing Home (Richmond B. Mowry)

PATIENT SERVICES

Audiometric and receptive communication screening

Individual patient screening report

Diagnostic hearing evaluation

Hearing-aid fitting

Hearing-aid evaluation

Hearing-aid repair

Hearing-aid maintenance program

Assistive listening devices: selection, fitting, and orientation

Cerumen management program

Direct consultation with residents, physicians, families, social workers, nursing staff, and significant others

Weekly in-house visits

Emergency service

FACILITY SERVICES

Ombudsman Reconciliation Act: Receptive communication classification of all new admissions—Minimum Data Sheet (MDS)

Patient-specific screening report for medical records

In-service training for nursing and administrative staff (continuing education unit [CEU]-approved)

In-service training for ancillary personnel (CEU-approved)

Americans with Disabilities Act (ADA) review and recommendations for compliance

Family night lecture series

SPECIAL SERVICES

Hospice patient care: Evaluations and loaner amplification devices (No charge to patients or nursing home facility.)

Medicaid patients not eligible for PETI (State funds): Amplification devices acquired through charity organizations

Hearing-aid safety cords for patients who cannot manage their own devices because of physical and/or mental conditions.

Chapter 8

Financial and Marketing Considerations in the Rehabilitation of Older Adults

Robert M. Traynor

The world is a cruel place. Hearing losses coexist in a world in which rents, taxes, equipment, employees, and other substantial expenses must be paid each month. In an audiology private practice, expenses and the clinician's own income depend on productivity—appropriate charges must be assessed for the practice to survive.

Most discussions of the financial aspects of providing hearing care to the elderly consist of lamentations regarding the lack of third-party payments. Indeed, there are real concerns among audiology practitioners regarding the lack of coverage of hearing aids and audiologic rehabilitation for the elderly from Medicare, Medicaid, and private insurance carriers. This chapter presents a perspective on financial issues in working with the elderly by focusing on the financial resources of this population. Rather than assuming that the elderly cannot afford audiologic services, the intent of this chapter is to discuss the resources that many elderly people in the 1990s do possess to pay for better hearing.

Audiologists donate too many services under the umbrella of being a helping profession. Most audiologists are educated in a well-meaning university program that emphasizes the helping aspects of the field but minimizes the realities of practice. This helping attitude is especially true in the profession's orientation toward providing services to the elderly population. In general, audiologists consider older patients as ones who do not have the resources to pay for hearing care. This was true of the elderly population in the 1960s and 1970s, but the financial composition of the elderly population has changed drastically over the past 10 to 20 years. In fact, one of the best kept secrets in the field is that older people are more capable now of purchasing products and services than they have been at any other time. For many economic reasons, such as changes in retirement dynamics, better planning, and better investment, the elders of the 1990s have the power to purchase health care services that are not covered by their insurance programs. The difficulties arise when patients present themselves as financially indigent but really have the ability to fund their hearing care. The purpose of this chapter is to present the information necessary to understand the real financial situation of older people and their ability to afford hearing care. An additional goal is to present marketing techniques to attract and retain older patients in an audiology practice.

WHAT DO THE ELDERLY BELIEVE?

Americans reflect on the 1990s as the era of the "me" generation. Much like the 1980s, the late 1910s and 1920s were a time of great affluence for Americans. Many people in the middle class considered themselves "rich" because of their savings, assets, or stock holdings. At the time of the stock market crash (October, 1929) and during the Great Depression, the current generation of elders were in their formative or young adult years. If they were not adults during the Depression, they were children who suffered the consequences of these times. It is difficult to imagine the frustration of elderly patients in the rough times of the 1930s. Our current elders or their parents were fired, companies went bankrupt, and banks closed owing millions to depositors. People who had been affluent became poor while the poor became destitute, and the financial habits of a generation of consumers were formed.

The unfortunate circumstances of a worldwide economic crisis in the 1930s produced a financially cautious generation of elderly consumers in the 1990s. This caution dominates the spending habits of these people. They postpone services they do not perceive as essential and attempt to purchase products and services at discount prices, even when they might be able to afford these items at a higher cost.

THE REAL FINANCIAL CONDITION OF ELDERLY PEOPLE

It is difficult to classify the financial condition of any diverse subgroup of the population, and extracting information from the overall data specifically about the elderly is a particularly difficult task. Some older people own their houses, can afford to travel, entertain friends, seek the best health care, and keep a presentable household and wardrobe. Others, however, barely exist on Social Security, pensions, investments, or their assets. To augment their incomes to meet expenses, the elderly often work. They earn extra income to facilitate retirement, and this activity complicates statistical investigation of the real incomes generated by the elderly population. The complications arise from substantial government incentive to elderly people not to report income earned. Retired wage-earners may be subject to a tax increase, and their wages may result in a reduction of their Social Security benefits. Because some older people underreport income obtained from earnings, assets, investments, and other sources, income statistics are not usually reflective of their true financial health. Similarly, older people often transfer title to much of their assets and investments to relatives while they are alive through a process termed *gifting*. Although gifting can save families large amounts of inheritance taxes, it compounds the difficulties encountered by statisticians attempting to accurately assess the income and true assets of the older population.

These concerns notwithstanding, the economic effects of aging are dynamic and seem to vary with overall worldwide economic conditions and the spending habits of particular generations of elders as well as government retirement and financial incentives. Economic changes occur slowly but substantially over long periods of time. For example, Atchley (1977) stated that in 1973, more than 50 percent of elderly white Americans were relatively poor and that 96 percent of black families had incomes that would classify them as poor. At that time, six of ten Americans were poor. Butler and Lewis (1977) indicated that the income levels used to estimate poverty during the 1970s were ridiculously low and that these figures drastically underestimated real poverty among older people. Thus, poverty in the 1970s was probably much greater than indicated by the literature.

Though the income levels at which poverty is officially declared are still unrealistic, Schulz (1992) stated that there has been a dramatic improvement in the financial plight of the elderly over the past decade. Rising Social Security incomes, private and government pensions, changing retirement patterns, and preparation for retirement have greatly reduced the dependency ratios for the elders of the 1990s compared with their counterparts in the 1960s and 1970s. Allen et al (1992) suggested that at present between 10 and 25 percent of the retired population older than 65 years still earn an income. When this income is considered, the poverty level for the elderly almost disappears.

The older population is more financially similar to the younger population than ever before. Schulz (1992) stated that among the elders of the 1990s there are some who are very rich, many with adequate incomes, many more with modest incomes (often near the unrealistic poverty level), and a large minority still destitute. It appears, however, that a large number of patients can afford audiologic services if the data generated by the United States Census (1990) in Figure 8–1 are considered. Even in the group 85 years of age and older, more than 20 percent of the population had an income greater than $30,000 with virtually no expenses other than health care. Although health care can be a substantial expense, a healthy older person can usually afford audiologic products and services.

In relation to purchasing power, discretionary income is of much greater interest than the overall income available to the elderly. Many healthy elderly people do not have high living expenses because the mortgage is often paid, the children have been reared, and most of the expenses of life have already been incurred. According to Allen et al (1992), a substantial proportion of

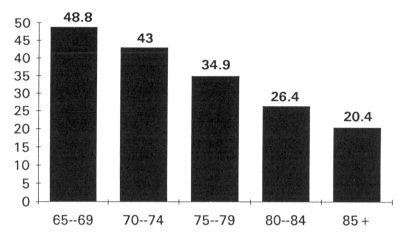

FIGURE 8–1   *Elderly with incomes greater than $30,000 (United States Census 1990).*

houses owned by the aged are mortgage-free. House ownership reduces the income needs of the aged in that normal costs and taxes are much less than the amount of rent required for comparable housing accommodations. It has been estimated that the maintenance costs for an unencumbered house are 30 to 40 percent less than the costs of renting comparable facilities. In addition, there is the possibility that the house can be used, in part, as an income-producing asset or that a home equity loan can be used to provide additional cash. Fisher (1992) indicated that the average household income peaks at $41,068 when the owners are between the ages of 45 and 54 years. Though average household income declines to $33,708 when the owners are 55 to 64 years of age and to $19,816 for owners older than 65 years, discretionary income continues to rise. People 65 years and older have the highest discretionary income of any age group (an average of $5,633) followed by the group 55 to 64 years of age ($4,906) and the group 45 to 54 years of age ($3,701). The United States Census Bureau (1990) reported that the group 65 years of age and older has more assets than younger groups and that their median net worth is twice as high as that of all households ($73,471 as opposed to $35,752).

These are only the reported figures. If older persons augment their incomes by working, the discretionary income is proportionally greater. In general, incomes among the elderly differ significantly among subgroups by variables such as age, sex, race, ethnicity, marital status, living arrangements, education, and former occupation. Although similar to other segments of the population in income, many elderly remain clustered just above the official poverty level and are extremely vulnerable to increasing health care costs.

Bodnar and Wilcox (1992) indicated that because of reduced consumer spending and overall improving economic conditions, people in the United States are in general more prosperous than in past years. The authors discussed the changes in prosperity according to the Kiplinger Personal Prosperity Index (KPI) for 1989 through 1991. The KPI considers all consumer items such as food, shelter, taxes, transportation, and other specific areas, and it indexes prosperity. The 1990 data indicated that prosperity decreased in 1990 in relation to 1989, whereas the 1991 data suggested that prosperity increased substantially in 1991 in relation to 1990. It should also be noted that prosperity according to the KPI increased for all age groups. In 1991 the prosperity indices for the groups 55 to 64 years of age and 65 years and older not only increased substantially over indices for 1989, but prosperity did not decrease for these groups in 1990 as much as it had for younger age groups. Although it took most of 1990 for people to pay off debts, Bodnar and Wilcox (1992) suggested that this increase in the KPI that began in 1991 will continue through the 1990s as all age groups begin to invest money rather than spend it.

Some patients truly have financial difficulties because of extremely high health care costs, particularly those with nursing home expenses. Nursing home and other major medical expenses can severely erode the principal of patients' investment assets, which are often used to provide a monthly income. To circumvent this disaster, an older couple in which one partner has a financial health care crisis can determine the net worth of their assets, and the incapacitated person becomes entitled to one-half of these assets. By law, once these assets are used, the incapacitated spouse becomes eligible for Medicaid to cover the health care expenses. The other partner uses the remaining assets for expenses, investments, and other purposes.

SOURCES OF INCOME

The Not-So-Fixed Income

Many patients in an audiology clinic refer to fixed incomes. They ask the audiologist, "That's a lot of money for a person on a fixed income. Don't you have a senior citizen's discount?" Although most clinicians are compassionate and try to accommodate patients who truly have minimal incomes or high health care expenses, Schulz (1992) indicated that older people with investments or property have the best edge against inflation of all segments of the population. These people have most of their funds invested, and the interest income usually rises and falls with the rate of inflation. Most pension programs, particularly the government plans, increase the retirement benefit for Cost of Living Allowances (COLA). The COLA, according to Allen et al (1992), is an adjustment in the retirement benefits (in theory, either an increase or a decrease) according to the Consumer Price Index or some other economic indicator. The philosophy behind the COLA is to assist the retiree in an adjustment for inflation, usually 3 to 4 percent per year. Because older people receive the COLA and interest on their invested funds and younger or working people may or may not receive a raise to offset increases in consumer prices, one could argue that people who have not retired may be receiving more of a fixed income than those who have retired.

Retirement Income

Many retirement plans are government-based systems, others are sponsored by private companies, and some are insurance or investment programs. Retirement planning is complicated by inflation, which can cause problems in predicting taxes and costs of living, such as food, extraneous expenses, and health care not covered by Medicare and the patient's supplemental plan. Figure 8–2 indicates the percentage of people in various age groups with income from reported earnings, interest, and retirement benefits. At the age of 55 years more than 91 percent of those polled during the 1990 United States Census were employed and earning an income. In contrast, only about 7 percent of those older than 85 years earned incomes.

According to the 1990 Census, one method of reporting investment income is as interest income. Note in Figure 8–2 that in the group as a whole, 70 percent of people received some sort of reported interest income when they were between the ages of 50 and 89 years. Though interest income is fairly constant over the age groups, retirement benefits for most people begin at the government-mandated 65 years of age. Interest from all sources and retirement benefits as presented in Figure 8–2 are the most important forms of overall income for the elderly. The United States Census (1990) also estimated that 36 percent of the population older then 65 years derive additional income from assets such as investment dividends, rental income from property, royalties, or estates and trusts. This percentage did not include people who derived income from wages earned.

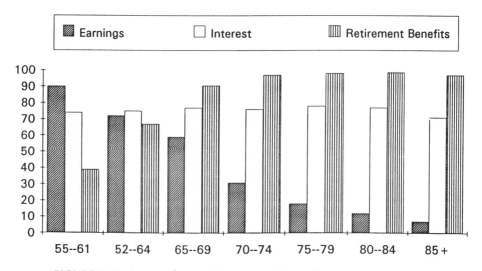

FIGURE 8–2   *Income from various sources (United States Census 1990).*

Benefits from sources other than Social Security that result in income to a retiree may be derived from a number of sources. The two most common types of non–Social Security income are public pension plans or private pension plans and annuities. The data on the number of people who receive retirement benefits from Social Security are compared with the data on the number of people who receive benefits from sources other than Social Security in Figures 8–3 and 8–4. Public pension incomes are received by people who held a position or occupation with the government or other public agency. An example of a public pension program (Figure 8–5) is military retirement. Similar to other public pension programs in general design, the military program is based on the grade at which the person retires and the number of years of service. In many public pension programs, medical care and other auxiliary benefits, such as commissary use, are included in the retirement benefit. Others that qualify as public pension plans are those that might be used by federal employees, railroad workers, or former state or municipal employees.

Private pensions or annuities are sponsored by private companies or often workers themselves. Though really a method of forced savings, some economists have suggested that private pension plans create a higher consumption level among the retired population and that these plans help maintain a high level of economic activity. Allen et al (1992) attributed the growth of private pensions to many factors, but the specific reasons for existence vary according to plan. In general, private pension plans seem to be motivated by employers attempting to increase worker productivity, succumbing to labor pressures, or attempting to decrease their tax burden. Because there

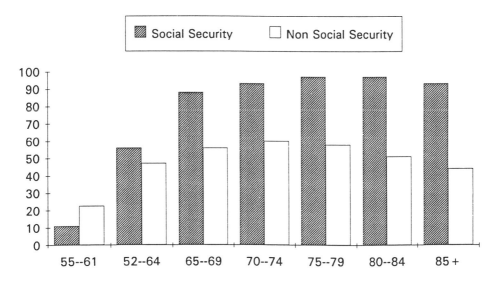

FIGURE 8–3   *Retirement benefits (United States Census 1990).*

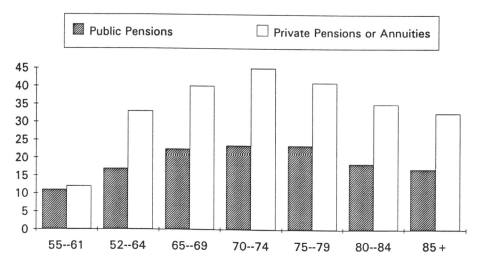

FIGURE 8–4   *Retirement benefits from sources other than Social Security (United States Census 1990).*

are so many different motivations for the establishment of these programs, it is difficult to characterize the private pension plans into a single philosophy or rationale. Although these programs were begun to reward workers for long periods of service, in recent years private pension plans have been modified to be deferred wages. This deferred wage concept views a pension benefit as part of a wage package that is composed of cash wages and other employee fringe benefits.

Whichever conceptual framework is considered, the burden of retirement security for elderly workers is spread over a large number of younger

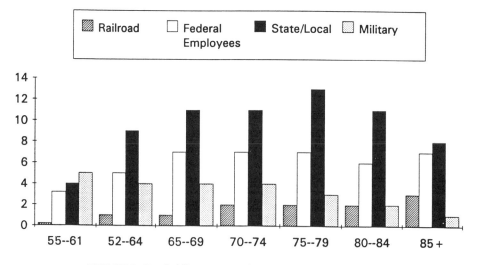

FIGURE 8–5   *Public pensions (United States Census 1990).*

workers over a long period of time. Benefits under these plans are highly variable and can often be obtained in addition to Social Security. Thus, some older patients have income from their private pension plans and from Social Security, securing a level of income comparable at retirement with that received as a worker.

Social Security

Hallman and Rosenbloom (1987) suggested that the Social Security system is considered one of the most complex and perplexing concepts ever designed, yet the basic philosophy is rather simple. The basis of Social Security is that during one's working years, employees, employers, and self-employed people pay Social Security taxes (Federal Insurance Contributions Act [FICA] taxes), which are pooled in special trust funds. When workers retire, die, or become disabled, monthly benefits are paid to the workers or their spouses to replace part of the lost earnings. Social Security eligibility is determined by the person's insured status. Eligibility for retirement and survivorship benefits generally requires that a worker, depending on the benefit sought, be fully insured or currently insured.

For most audiology patients, fully insured status involves working in an environment that covers workers for Social Security over 40 quarters. Some may obtain eligibility for benefits by working at least one quarter for every calendar year since 1950 (or after the year in which they turned 21 years of age, if later) up to the year they reach 62 years of age, die, or become disabled. In any case, a minimum of six quarters is required before any benefits can be authorized under the Social Security system. Currently insured status is used, according to Hallman and Rosenbloom (1987), to qualify for survivor benefits under the system and is achieved when the worker has been credited with a minimum of six quarters of coverage during the 13-quarter period ending with the quarter in which he or she died.

The benefits of a Social Security retirement include a monthly income that begins as a full benefit at a specified retirement age, somewhere between 65 and 67 years depending on the year that the retired worker reaches 62 years of age and continues from the specified full benefit retirement age for the remainder of the retired person's lifetime. There are reduced retirement benefits for early retirement between the ages of 62 years and full-benefit retirement age. The amount of the monthly benefit is determined by a formula based on the worker's covered earnings over the working years less any deductions for early retirement. The spouse (or divorced spouse, if the marriage existed for at least 10 years immediately before the divorce) of a retired worker is entitled to a benefit, called the spousal benefit. The spousal benefit is equal to 50 percent of the worker's benefit, if the spouse is 65 years of age (the present full-benefit retirement) or older. Although Social Security benefits are partially or fully income tax–free, the total of all Social Security retirement benefits is subject to an overall family maximum. The maximum family benefit (MFB) is applicable when more than two beneficiaries are receiving benefits on the same earnings record (ie, a retired worker and two or more auxiliary beneficiaries).

A patient who is retired under the Social Security system has specific restrictions on the amount of income that he or she may earn and remain eligible for full retirement benefits. The government's method of restricting this income is the retirement earnings test. Myers (1992) stated that the underlying principle of the retirement earnings test is that retirement benefits should be paid only to those who are substantially retired. Full Social Security benefits are paid to retirees if their earnings do not exceed the annual exemption amount. These exemptions change periodically according to law and also vary according to the retiree's age. Currently, for a retired person younger than 65 years who earns more than the exemption amount ($7,440), for every $2.00 earned in income, $1.00 of retirement benefit is withheld. For a person older than 65 years but younger than 70 years, the exemption is $10,200, and $1.00 for every $3.00 of income is withheld. Though discouraged, after 70 years of age a retiree may earn income above the exemption amount without any reduction in retirement benefit.

Investments

Schulz (1992) stated that most older people have a large measure of protection from inflation because of their investments, such as certificates of deposit (CDs), mutual funds, and other financial devices. In the early 1980s, most banks were lending their consumers money at 25 percent interest. These institutions obtained their funds from elderly people who invested in a CD or other investments. During this time, investors could receive a substantial return on their investment, at the expense of bank customers who could not afford a business loan or to buy a house because of high interest rates. Because they invest much more of their money than do younger people, older people received a bonanza in interest income at that time. Though the 1990s show promise for low interest rates and low inflation, Schulz (1992) suggested that older people have more of a hedge on inflation because of the nature of various investment opportunities. Some of these investments offer users some risk (Figure 8–6). The bottom of the pyramid suggests relatively safe investments, and the peak of the pyramid indicates extremely risky investments. As the investor proceeds from safe investments to investments of increased risk, the chance for loss of the principal increases. Conversely, as the investor proceeds from risky investments to safe ones, the chance that the funds invested will lose purchasing power increases. Most patients who seek audiologic services have investments within the first row of Figure 8–6 and life insurance because these investments have the least risk of loss of investment principal and often provide income.

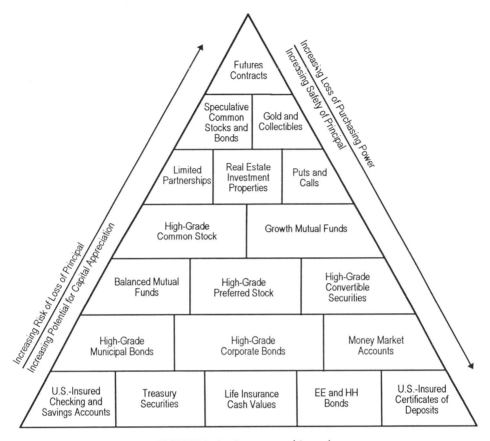

FIGURE 8–6   *Investment hierarchy*

(Reprinted with permission from Certified Financial Planning Course 1991)

Certificates of Deposit

Although they allow the lowest return of most securities, CDs (see Figure 8–6) yield a known interest rate if kept until maturity. According to Mayo (1991), a federally insured CD has almost no risk of default by the bank in its payment of principal and interest. Essentially if a person holds a certificate until maturity, money is paid back with the negotiated interest rate for the use of the funds during the agreed time. Perceived as the safest type of investment, CDs are popular, especially with elderly investors. On occasion, a patient who has a CD may need to postpone payment for services or products until the CD accrues full interest at maturity.

Life Insurance

Life insurance is another investment used by all age groups because it may serve a dual purpose—provision of a death benefit and investment. Life insurance commonly comes in one of three forms—term, whole life, or endowment—or a combination of two or more of the three.

Term insurance provides financial protection for a specified period. If death occurs during this period, the face amount of the policy is paid to the beneficiary, and nothing paid if the insured person survives the policy period. Term insurance can be compared with other forms of insurance, such as property insurance, in that it does not accrue cash or loan values.

Whole-life policies provide protection for the entire life of the insured regardless of how many years premiums are paid. Whole-life policies require the payment of a premium throughout the insured's lifetime or over a limited period, such as 10, 20, or 30 years. These policies accrue cash values and loan values through an excess of premiums in the early years of the policy and through compounded interest. This is the investment portion of the whole-life insurance policy.

Endowments pay the face value of the policy in a fixed period, such as 10, 25, or 30 years. They are savings plans with a life-insurance benefit element.

Annuities

Annuities involve a contractual arrangement that assures a person an income that he or she cannot outlive as well as an income that is relatively large compared with the amount paid for the annuity. The periodic income under the annuity should be relatively large because the annuity principal involves the gradual consumption of the purchase price of the annuity. The investor, in deciding which route to take, should evaluate payments under annuity against the return rate from relatively safe CDs or high-yield municipal, corporate, or government bonds.

An annuity can be purchased with a single premium or paid over a period of years to retirement. If the annuitant dies before 65 years of age (or other selected maturity date), the contract provides for the payment of the accumulated gross premiums (without interest) or the cash value, whichever is larger, as a death benefit to the beneficiary designated in the contract. Premiums for annuities are usually quoted on the basis that the accumulated sum at maturity will be applied under a life annuity with 120 or 240 monthly installments guaranteed. At maturity the annuitant may elect any form of life annuity and the actual monthly income is appropriately adjusted. In addition, the annuitant usually has the option of taking the accumulated contract value in cash instead of in the form of an annuity. This can often be a valuable option, because it may be in the annuitant's best interest to cash in and reinvest in a vehicle that brings a higher return.

Government Securities

Many types of debt securities are issued by federal agencies and by federal, state, and local governments. United States Treasury securities are issued to help finance the federal government. Although treasury securities and series EE and HH bonds are considered risky, they are relatively safe from default because of the credit worthiness of the federal government. Another attractive feature of treasury securities and other government securities is that the interest income is exempt from state and local income taxes. Government securities include different types of municipal, state, and federal bonds that also facilitate a tax-exempt return at relatively low risk. Although these investments appear safe and attractive to the investor, they should be considered long-term investments. Thus they represent a risk of loss of purchasing power of the principal used in the investment.

Mutual Funds

Mutual funds can be divided into two groups—income or growth—depending on the objective. The objective of an income fund is to provide income for the investor. The goal of a growth fund is the growth of capital or appreciation of the principal invested. There are many types of funds in each category, and elderly patients may have some of each type. The investments in the other rows of Figure 8–6 are often part of mutual funds, in which a group of investors hires a manager to invest their money for them. In a mutual fund, investors who share a common goal (income or growth) and who are limited in time and investment resources, pool their funds to purchase securities to meet these common financial objectives. Each investor owns a number of shares in the investments conducted by the money manager. The value of the fund increases or decreases with the success of the investments made by the money manager.

Older people usually do not invest in speculative investments such as futures contracts or other extremely risky ventures. On occasion, to obtain a higher return on their investment (and thus more income), they might participate in a mutual fund that invests in some of these risky ventures as part of its overall portfolio. The advantages of these shared-risk ventures is that if the fund chooses an investment that is not doing well, it is often averaged into other better investments, and the overall effect of a bad investment by the fund is substantially reduced to the individual investor. Thus, for the elderly these investments are a relatively safe place to store money, either for growth or to provide primary or supplemental income.

More than 70 percent of the elderly interviewed in the 1990 United States Census received interest income (Figure 8–2), most likely from a combination of the aforedescribed investments. This income may be in addition to Social Security benefits, private pension benefits, or another retirement program. Clinicians must be sensitive to patients who are truly indigent while simultaneously offering audiologic products and services at a fair price. As they offer their services, clinicians must realize that older patients often have more resources than are readily apparent, particularly in the 1990s.

MARKETING AUDIOLOGY TO THE ELDERLY

Marketing is relatively new to audiologists. Until recently, audiologists had not advertised their abilities, skills, products, and procedures to patients who were prospects for audiologic services. Aggressive marketing of products and services to the public is relatively new to audiology and other medical services. In the early days of the profession, there were few trained professionals to provide audiologic services, and competition was minimal. Recently, particularly in places where it is desirable to live, the competition has become substantial and has produced the need for aggressive marketing. Competition for patients with hearing impairments exists among audiologists, otolaryngologists, and hearing-aid dealers. The wise businessperson must present his or her practice as unique from the competition. Although marketing is labor intensive, it is impossible to provide the best in hearing care and products if the patients do not come to the clinic for treatment. With successful marketing, patients will seek assistance and they will seek it at a particular clinic.

The Basics

First, the successful marketing of an audiology practice to any population, especially the elderly, involves five essential components: market research, product development, distribution, pricing, and promotion. If these fundamentals are not considered, a new practice will have serious growing pains and will often not be successful.

A market survey determines if the products and services considered are needed within a certain geographic market area. The survey may determine whether the practice has too much competition for one particular age group or for certain products, such as hearing aids. The survey may suggest specific techniques, services, or products to attract a certain market. A practice should not be opened in a particular geographic area until a positive market survey is obtained.

Product development is the specific orientation of products and services toward certain consumer demands identified in the marketing survey. If the competition is keen, development of a unique product identification for the practice may be necessary. Product identification includes tailoring the practice to meet unmet needs identified in the marketing survey, such as professional services not being offered at present, high-technology products, better office hours, more convenient location, or office aesthetics.

The method of distribution of products and services must be determined. For most clinics, the method of distribution is at the professional retail level, selling the products for suggested retail prices and offering services for the usual and customary fees in the geographic area.

The two areas of marketing that are important once the other aspects have been considered are pricing and promotion. Affixing a price to a service or a product should involve not only evaluation of what the competition charges for the service but also calculation of the overhead expenses of the new clinic to offer the service or the product. Expenses such as salary, taxes, commissions, equipment, repairs, rent, telephone, travel, cost of products, office supplies, clinical supplies, attorneys, accountants, and advertising must be considered as part of the fee structure in the computation of retail prices for products such as hearing instruments and assistive devices.

Promotion of the successful practice should be directed not only to elderly hearing-aid users but also to physicians of various specialties. Providing a variety of services, including audiometric evaluations, audiologic rehabilitation, electrophysiologic evaluations, and tests for neural integrity aid in marketing. Successful practitioners realize that the elderly are an important portion of their business, and these clients must be attracted to the clinic.

Specific Promotion to the Elderly

Because the audiologic services used by the elderly are dispensing of hearing aids and audiologic rehabilitation, the marketing of these services to the elderly is extremely important. Promotional endeavors by audiologists have been assisted by market analysis. Kochkin (1993b) suggested that the market for potential users of hearing aids is primarily people 45 years of age and older. In his MarkeTrak III Survey, Kochkin investigated why people with hearing losses do not own hearing devices. The reasons cited were as follows:

- Hearing instruments have a stigma attached to them
- The person's hearing loss is not serious enough to warrant hearing instruments
- Hearing instruments are uncomfortable or do not perform well
- Hearing instruments cost too much, especially in relation to their value

Could these problem areas be used in advertising products and procedures? Advertisements for small hearing aids show young people in the advertisements who are active and happy. Other advertisements discuss hearing in background noise and other problems. For years, professionals who advertise hearing aids have successfully catered to these perceived difficulties.

Kochkin's (1993a,b) data can be used to target patients by age group and by their potential benefits from certain products. Schweitzer (1986) suggested that a good salesperson helps a customer discover the value of the hearing aid (or hearing-care services) by repeating to the client situational comments heard during the interview. The marketing effort should assist elderly patients in overcoming the various reasons for not owning hearing instruments. Kochkin (1992) organized factors that influence first-time buyers of hearing instruments (Table 8–1). These items are the reasons that motivated patients to seek assistance for their hearing impairment. Physicians recommended a substantial number of the hearing aids purchased. Thus, the successful marketing of a practice must include good referral relations with the medical community. Family members influence the motivation of a patient to seek assistance. All other advertising, according to Kochkin's data, is secondary to the physician, the family, and other professional recommendations. Advertising to the family and to physicians is a practice-builder because these groups exert substantial influence on an elderly person's motivation to seek hearing care. Once the patient has made the decision to seek assistance for the hearing impairment, clinicians must influence the situation with advertising to ensure they, and not a competitor, receive the referral.

Promotion of the practice must establish the proper image in the minds of prospective patients and their families. A practice interested in hearing care for the elderly must be selective in the marketing conducted, its presentation, and the personnel who represent the practice to facilitate the correct perception of the practice. Staab (1985) suggested various types of personalities among the hearing-impaired community. Of the types who seek audiologic services or products for hearing loss, some are interested in technology, others in the aesthetics of the clinic, brand-name products, or other considerations. The elderly and their families, however, are usually interested in finding a clinic that is stable and that offers the security of personable, qualified audiologists. They desire hearing care provided by someone who is

TABLE 8–1   Factors That Influence First-time Users of Hearing Aids

Factor	1989	1990	1991
Hearing loss got worse	72.2	69.3	55.8
Hearing loss literature	10.5	9.1	2.0
Better Hearing Institute	2.0	1.7	0
Advertisement in magazine	4.0	1.4	2.0
Advertisement in newspaper	2.5	5.6	4.0
Advertisement on television	6.5	3.6	4.5
Ear doctor	28.6	33.7	19.1
Family doctor	17.2	18.7	7.0
Audiologist	25.7	34.9	26.6
Hearing-aid specialist	15.9	14.3	14.1
Family members	52.2	54.6	56.8
Boss or co-worker	3.2	1.6	4.5
Industry celebrity	3.3	3.8	0.5
Direct mail	2.9	3.2	2.5
Telemarketing phone call	0.7	0.9	0

(Reprinted with permission from Kochkin 1992)

knowledgeable and has been in practice for a number of years, because this quality ensures a high level of continuous care and service.

Because many elderly patients are handicapped to some degree, accommodation to various handicapping conditions should be an integral component of the clinic, the clinical services offered, and the overall marketing plan for attracting the elderly. Many elderly people are handicapped by difficulties that limit their transportation and ambulation. They may be interested in receiving clinical services close to their residence or from a clinic that accommodates their transportation needs. Handicapped patients may have to rely on friends, relatives, and others to transport them to the clinic. Some patients must use public transportation if they do not have friends who drive or close relatives or if they cannot afford a caretaker. The practice location should be accessible to public transportation and perhaps offer some reimbursement for fares. The clinic itself should be accessible to the handicapped in the design of its doors, hallways, and parking, including ramps where necessary. Home services are an integral part of providing hearing care to the elderly and handicapped.

Overall, the older public perceives most hearing aids as essentially the same, and often shops for these products. Most can probably afford hearing care, but the elderly are not particularly impressed with recent advances in technology unless they have had difficulties with their current instruments. Patients who have had difficulty with hearing instruments often shop for technology but do not understand it. For example, they may think that a single-amplifier *bill*-circuited device is the same as a two-amplifier *pill* circuit for hundreds less in cost. The elderly do not understand why hearing aids cost more than they think they should, because of the economic beliefs discussed earlier. It is often necessary for the audiologist to conduct demonstrations to present the benefits of the true differences in technology.

The marketing of an audiology practice to the elderly consists of sound marketing techniques specifically tuned to the elderly population of a particular geographic area. It involves catering to this population by advertising, soliciting recommendations from physicians, and sound rehabilitative techniques that use state-of-the-art products. Important to success is the personality of the clinician as well as location and other factors. Rehabilitative treatment of the elderly is a professionally and economically rewarding endeavor, but obtaining new patients each year in a competitive environment should be an ongoing process.

REFERENCES

Allen, E.T., Melone, J.J., Rosenbloom, J.S., & VanDerhei, J.L. (1992). *Pension planning* (7th ed), Homewood: Irwin.

Atchley, R.C. (1977). *The social forces in later life* (2nd ed.), Belmont: Wadsworth.

Bodnar, J., & Wilcox, M.D. (1992). Cheer up America. *Kiplinger Personal Finance Magazine, 46,* pp. 71-75.

Butler, R.N., & Lewis, M.I. (1977). *Aging and mental health* (2nd ed.), St. Louis: Mosby.

Certified Financial Planning Course (1991). *Investments* (Study Guide No. 3). Denver: College for Financial Planning.

Fisher, C. (1992). Boomers bringing buying power. *Advertising Age. November 16,* pp. 14-17.

Hallman, V.G., & Rosenbloom, J.S. (1987). *Personal financial planning* (4th ed.). St. Louis: McGraw-Hill.

Kochkin, S. (1992). MarkeTrak III: Higher hearing aid sales don't signal better market penetration. *Hearing Journal, 45,* 47-54.

Kochkin, S. (1993a). MarkeTrak III: Why 20 million in US don't use hearing aids for their hearing loss, *Hearing Journal, 46,* 20-27.

Kochkin, S. (1993b). MarkeTrak III: Why 20 million in US don't use hearing aids for their hearing loss, *Hearing Journal, 46,* 26-31.

Mayo, H.B. (1991). *Investments: An introduction.* Chicago: Dryden. Myers, R.J. (1992). Social security and Medicare. In J.S. Rosenbloom (Ed.), *The handbook on employee benefits* (3rd ed.) pp. 154-157. Homewood: Business One Irwin.

Schulz, J.H. (1992). *The economics of aging* (5th ed.). New York: Auburn.

Schweitzer, H.C. (1986). Reflections on the significance of private practice dispensing. *Seminars in Hearing, 7,* 205-212.

Staab, W.J. (1985). Marketing. Presented at Jackson Hole Rendezvous Hearing Health Conference, August 30-September 3, 1985, Jackson Hole, Wyo.

United States Bureau of the Census, Current Population Reports (1990). Money income of persons by level and median income, Document 729, Washington: United States Government Printing Office.

Chapter 9

Group Hearing Care for Older Adults

Sharon A. Lesner

Group treatment is an excellent medium for providing audiologic rehabilitation. The essence of all groups, formal or informal, is that they revolve around communication among members (Barr, 1988). There is no better mode to provide opportunities for practice, teaching, and modification of communicative behaviors. In addition, programs that focus on self-help and education also provide attention to the psychosocial changes that result from disabilities. These programs can, as a result, aid older people in leading more satisfying lives (Kemp, 1990). The purpose of this chapter is to explore the opportunities provided by group hearing care. Suggestions concerning factors that influence the success of group work are provided with a description of a model hearing-aid orientation program for older adults and their significant others.

Considering the low rates of satisfaction reported by new users of hearing aids who do not receive organized postfitting sessions (Brooks, 1979, 1985; Kapteyn, 1977; Surr et al, 1978; Ward & Gowers, 1980), audiologic rehabilitation should be available for all people who obtain hearing aids, especially older adults. It is not enough to instruct the person to "call me if you have a problem" (Hickson et al, 1986; Rubinstein & Cherry, 1988). Hearing aids must be provided as part of a comprehensive program of audiologic rehabilitation. Groups provide an excellent method for providing the needed training and for helping to ensure quality hearing care.

ADVANTAGES OF GROUP WORK

Group work can be efficient and cost effective for providing audiologic rehabilitation. There are several advantages that result from group work for the person who is hearing impaired, the significant other, and the practitioner.

Advantages for the Person with the Hearing Impairment

In content, group work facilitates the rehabilitative process with repeated learning and problem-solving opportunities. Nearly 30 percent of wearers of hearing aids stop using the hearing aid, usually within the first 3 months (Brooks, 1985; Ross, 1987). The primary reason for discontinuing the use of hearing aids is that people do not know how to manage them (Kapteyn, 1977). Group work provides opportunities to identify and overcome problems that most commonly lead to discontinuation of the use of amplification. Montgomery (1991) suggested that group participation is the best insurance that hearing aids will be worn.

Hearing aids are only a part of the rehabilitative process. The roles of assistive listening devices (ALDs), audiovisual speech reception, and communication strategies in improving communication also need to be explored and optimized.

Although content-related information is important, group participation can provide substantial psychosocial benefits. In particular, realistic expectations can be developed, support can be drawn from members (especially in the realization that there are others with similar problems), and ventilation of feelings can result. Group interactions can reduce feelings of isolation and aid in the development of self-confidence. Both content and emotional support counseling can be provided.

Group work with people who do not wear hearing aids also can be productive (Hardick & Lesner, 1979). People who do not wear aids can be helped in overcoming denial by associating with and benefiting from the peer support of successful wearers. Opportunities to try hearing aids and ALDs during the sessions may demonstrate the advantages of amplification. People who do not wear hearing aids can be taught to maximize communication through the appropriate use of communication strategies and environmental engineering and manipulation.

Advantages for Significant Others

The greatest enemy of people with hearing impairments is often the people who love them most, namely their significant others. Significant others usually do not have an accurate understanding of the problems associated with hearing loss, and they often have unrealistic expectations of the person with the hearing impairment and of the hearing aids. It is not unusual, for example, for significant others to expect that the use of a hearing aid cures the hearing loss or that attendance at speechreading classes enables people with hearing impairments to speechread perfectly. Providing significant others with knowledge of the consequences of hearing loss and with training in how to maximize communication can be beneficial. Emotional issues related to the hearing loss and the consequences of the loss can be addressed during group sessions. Participants can benefit from knowing that there are others who are experiencing problems caused by the presence of a hearing impairment, and people with hearing impairments and significant others benefit from the input provided by others.

Because communication between people with hearing impairments and significant others represents the most important communication dyad, both people need to be involved in the rehabilitative process. Audiologists should work to develop and reinforce effective communication behaviors and eliminate nonproductive behaviors.

Practitioner Advantages

Providing group services can be a source of professional satisfaction, especially when orchestrated appropriately. It is a gratifying experience to deliver high-quality services to patients and their significant others. Developing rapport with patients provides insights as to the efficacy of services, feedback concerning fitting protocols, information about the quality and workmanship of hearing aids and ALDs, insights about the problems experienced by people with hearing impairments, successful communication strategies, and research opportunities. The good will that is established between patients and practitioner often translates into referrals, and ultimately financial reward. Sales of ALDs are also more likely as a result of providing rehabilitative services.

MAXIMIZING GROUP WORK

Planning can maximize the effectiveness of group work. Important factors to consider include the need to establish the purpose of the group, publicize the group, compose the group, finance the group, prepare and orient members, and prepare the environment (Toseland, 1990).

Purpose of Hearing-Care Groups

Group work with older adults has been growing steadily in popularity and is being used in a wide variety of settings with various formats (Toseland, 1990). The structure of a group can be used to emphasize content goals or counseling. Regardless of the orientation, all groups have both content and socioemotional needs, and both types of needs must be met if the group is to be successful. Older adults tend to value groups in which attention is paid to their socioemotional needs, even at the expense of task accomplishment (Toseland, 1990).

The particular orientation of this chapter is on groups designed to restore, maintain, and enhance the function of older people with hearing impairments. Specific goals and activities are suggested at the end of the chapter. In addition to areas the clinician plans to include, it is wise to seek input from group members concerning areas on which they would like to focus. The benefits of this preparation include making the sessions relevant, inclusion of the members, and the development of a sense of group ownership. Such preparation also provides an efficient use of time for the participants.

Publicizing and Marketing the Group

Practitioners may need to publicize to enlist members for a new group. Audiologists, physicians, and speech-language pathologists may be a source of referrals. Other strategies and sources may yield members. Colleagues within one's own practice setting are a good source with which to begin. Making group participation a mandatory part of hearing-aid dispensing is an excellent approach to quality hearing care.

It may be necessary to publicize the availability of the group to colleagues in the area. This can be done with letters, newsletters, meetings, electronic-mail, press releases, newspaper and newsletter stories, and radio and television advertisements or announcements.

In the community, signs, notices in bulletins (eg, church, library) and newsletters and talks to senior groups can be productive. In Akron, the listing of senior groups is 20 pages long. Groups are usually anxious to have speakers, and this provides an excellent opportunity to make oneself known and to publicize one's program. The groups may also be interested in hearing screenings.

With the high prevalence of hearing loss, screening older adults can provide an extensive list of potential participants. During one screening I conducted in a senior center, for example, 204 people were tested and 199 did not pass the screening test. The information from the audiograms and the group sessions were explained to these people, and several groups were formed. Because of the large numbers of people involved, it was possible to compose groups of people who were experiencing similar hearing problems.

Other possibilities for identifying participants include visiting areas, programs, and places associated with older adults. These may include programs for people 65 years and older, senior centers, age-segregated housing, churches, adult education programs, social service agencies, consumer organizations, and college reunions.

Composing and Preparing the Group

It is necessary to decide if the group is to be open or closed to new members. The positive aspect of an open group is that with ongoing programming, individual members can participate in missed sessions or repeat sessions as needed. Adding new members, however, tends to alter group dynamics. When individual members miss sessions, they do not have the same common understanding and shared experiences as others. The advantage of closed membership is the development of cohesion and camaraderie (Toseland, 1990).

The optimum size of a group is six to ten members. This number might include three to five dyads between people with hearing impairments and their significant others. This size allows for optimum participation by group members without their feeling pressured to participate. The number should be adjusted upward or downward based on the degree of handicap experienced by the participants and the number of professional staff members participating.

The type and degree of hearing loss and the presence of other related handicaps should be considered when composing groups. Group members should be homogenous in degree and duration of hearing loss. People with similar hearing losses typically experience similar difficulties, so the focus of the group sessions can be narrowed. Special groups composed of people with Meniere syndrome, unilateral losses, severe to profound losses, and poor speech discrimination may be developed so that the unique problems associated with these losses can be effectively handled. When the pool of potential participants is low, it is possible to run groups with people from different socioeconomic and cultural groups. Speech discrimination ability should, however, be similar.

Contraindications to group participation include the presence of cognitive impairments, depression, or severe health problems. The presence of these problems can limit or disrupt participation. In these cases, the clinician should focus on the significant others, who should be taught how to manage the amplification devices. Visual status must be considered, especially if written evaluations are given or group speechreading tests or speech discrimination tests are to be administered. Other practical problems that may limit or preclude participation include transportation and scheduling difficulties. Older adults tend to have myriad activities, including vacations, that make scheduling difficult. In fact, open groups are often necessary to accommodate the scheduling conflicts.

Financing the Group

Financing group work varies with the facility or practitioner offering the services. Determination of costs and fees for group work and obtaining payment can be difficult and complex. It would seem that to calculate costs, the hourly fee should be divided by the number of group members. Several complications exist, however. Groups tend to last longer than individual therapy, and administrative costs remain the same per person. Groups may involve costs for publicity and marketing, preparation time, and materials. Adding additional paid staff also increases costs (Rose, 1989).

Options for financing group work include charging a fee for the cost of the service, including the fee in the cost of a hearing aid, or obtaining grants from outside agencies such as trust funds, foundations, corporations, and not-for-profit service groups (Fisher & Games, 1993). Clients tend to be reluctant to pay for rehabilitation services in advance. Some practitioners ask for a voluntary payment after the sessions are completed or ask patients to pay for the sessions on the basis of perceived worth. Philosophically and economically, the last two alternatives are not recommended.

Other possibilities include financing the sessions through tuition-based university or community college continuing education programs. The University of Akron, for example, offers a "60 Plus" program in which older people can enroll, without a fee, in college courses. Although the audiology department may not receive fees directly from such a source, it does benefit from subvention. Bally and Kaplan (1988) offered hearing rehabilitation programs through the Elderhostel program.

Sessions may be considered a business investment. The benefits to the patient and the practice may not be totally monetary. The reduction in the number of trouble-shooting visits and returned hearing aids can be considerable. In addition, the good will that results when patients understand the use of their hearing aids, when they use and are satisfied with the devices, and when they are convinced that the audiologist is concerned about their welfare is the best advertisement any practice can have. Unhappy hearing-aid consumers seem to talk to more people about their situation than satisfied hearing-aid wearers. Satisfied wearers of hearing aids are an excellent referral source.

Preparing and Orientating Members

Group members should be contacted before the first session with a letter or telephone call or during a clinic visit. Potential members should be provided with information concerning the purpose and potential benefits of the group. A description of when and where the groups are held and information about any related costs should be supplied. If they are to be included, significant others should be invited at this time. It is helpful to emphasize that the sessions will be fun as well as beneficial. Potential members should be encouraged to attend, even if they are not sure. The most difficult aspect of group work is usually getting the members in the door the first time. Mentioning that coffee and food will be provided can help to motivate some people.

Preparing the Environment

Because older adults experience sensory changes as they age and they may also have chronic disabilities, the environment in which group work is conducted should be carefully considered. Good environmental design can improve both rehabilitative interactions and outcomes (Hiatt, 1990); bad environmental design can limit effectiveness. Physical environment and psychosocial environment should be considered.

Physical Environment

The acoustic environment must be a prime focus for those who provide audiologic rehabilitation. In addition to minimizing ambient noise, ALDs should be used to improve the signal-to-noise ratio (S/N). Systems such as frequency modulation (FM), loops, or public address systems may be especially beneficial.

The visual environment should be designed to optimize communication and comfort. Sufficient nondirectional light should be provided, and sources of glare should be eliminated. Several of the visual changes that occur with age result in a need for greater illumination to optimize visual input (see Chapter 1).

Seating arrangements should ensure that participants are close to and at appropriate angles to the professional staff and other participants. Sitting at tables tends to reduce intimacy, increase the distance between participants, and produce poor angles for speechreading purposes. Placing chairs in a semicircle can minimize these problems. If a hard surface is needed on which to write or if refreshments are served, a round table should be used. If more than one professional is involved, the staff members should sit among the group members. In this way, visual and acoustic input to the members is maximized and the professionals can assist members who are on either side of them. The professionals should try to sit next to the people with the greatest difficulty. An assistant should be provided for people who need help with writing or who have visual problems. For the latter, the assistant can aid the person with the visual impairment and provide needed descriptions. Table 9–1 lists several factors to consider when selecting the site for group sessions. The key factor is accessibility.

TABLE 9–1 Considerations in Site Selection for Group Work

Sufficient space

Accessibility to people with handicaps

Low ambient noise

Nonskid carpeting as opposed to scatter rugs

Comfortable temperature

Adequate ventilation

Sufficient lighting with no glare

No distractions

Appropriate acoustic environment

Large easy-to-read signs posted at eye level

Parking

Seating that provides support and is easy to lower oneself onto and rise from

Psychosocial Environment

The professional and support staff of the facility in which the group sessions are offered must have positive attitudes concerning the potential of older patients. If negative attitudes are present, the best technical skills and intervention are not sufficient to provide a positive outcome. In fact, rehabilitative success or failure is rarely due to the lack of technical skill of the professionals delivering the treatment (Kemp, 1990). Instead, several important psychosocial factors influence the ultimate outcome for both the professional and the patient.

The professional staff must have positive attitudes concerning a patient's potential to have improved function, independence, life satisfaction, and self-esteem (Kemp, 1990). The staff cannot harbor ageist attitudes. An attitude of devaluation (Vash, 1981) often exists toward adults. With devaluation, a person is seen as less valuable, less attractive, less desirable, or less acceptable than someone else. Devaluation is a common reaction to older people, especially people with disabilities. Rehabilitative efforts will not be successful unless the staff believes that success is possible. The self-fulfilling prophecy does exist and can permeate the entire operation of a program.

Attention to the psychosocial changes that occur among people as a result of disability is also important. Key elements associated with the outcome of rehabilitative intervention are the motivation, cognitive ability, depressive state, and personality traits of the patient (Kemp, 1990). Factors such as passivity, dependence, antisocial behavior, histrionics, or suspicion are not conducive to rehabilitative success (Kemp, 1990).

There are several positive predictors of rehabilitative success. The positive indicators include the presence of assertiveness, close involvement with at least one other person on an intimate basis, and the ability to focus on life goals (Table 9–2).

GROUP LEADERSHIP

Group leadership is probably the key to success in group work. Because rehabilitation is as much a philosophy as it is a set of procedures, the interests, attitudes, and experience of the leader are extremely important. The leader

TABLE 9–2   Considerations for Scheduling Group Work

Avoid scheduling sessions at night, because of fear of crime and increased difficulty driving in darkness because of vision problems

Consider availability of transportation, including bus service and availability of significant others

Schedule sessions at times other than rush hour

Provide sessions during various times of the year to minimize difficulties due to winter weather, vacations, or holiday activities sets the tone for the group. In fact, a successful professional-patient relationship is paramount to effective hearing care (Clark, 1994).

There are several desirable characteristics of group leaders; these characteristics include both skills and personal qualities. Knowledge of the subject is important, and being a good speaker is helpful. Simple actions such as speaking loudly and slowly, not omitting words, pronouncing words carefully, avoiding behaviors such as pacing the room, putting hands in front of the mouth, and chewing or putting things in the mouth, as well as facing the group at an optimum vertical (not more than 30 degrees) and horizontal angle (not more than 45 degrees) can greatly facilitate communication. Highlighting important information can aid in teaching.

Several personal qualities are needed. These include empathy, genuineness, respect, and a true interest in and care about people. Empathy is basic to all helping relationships (Brammer, 1981). Empathy consists of putting oneself in the other person's place and seeing the world the way the other person sees it. Genuineness or congruence implies that one acts like oneself and does not put on airs. In a genuine person, acts and attitudes match. Warmth and caring are difficult to describe and quantify; however, behaviors such as smiling, making eye contact, touching, paying attention, and exercising courtesy all contribute.

Several other qualities contribute to success when working with older adults. Corey and Corey (1977) cite the following qualities as being important:

A genuine respect for older people

A history of positive experiences with older adults

A deep sense of caring for the elderly

An ability and desire to learn from the elderly

An understanding of the biologic aspects of aging

The conviction that the last years of life can be challenging

Patience, especially with repetition of stories

Knowledge of the special biologic, psychologic, and social needs of the aged

Sensitivity to the burdens and anxieties of the old

The ability to encourage older people to challenge many of the myths about old age

A healthy attitude regarding one's own eventual old age

A group leader can facilitate group function in a number of ways. Nonverbal behaviors such as body position, frequent eye contact, and gestures and verbal statements can indicate that the leader hears and understands what group members are saying (Roberts & Bouchard, 1989). Hellos and goodbyes are important. The goodbye provides an opportunity for the practitioner to pass along individualized information and suggestions. Appropriate touching and closeness and sincere praise, compliments, and use of names are beneficial. Using the first name can lessen the formality of the group; however, older people may believe it shows a lack of respect. Ask for each member's preference.

The amount that can be accomplished, especially in individual work done in conjunction with group work, can be increased if co-leaders or other professional staff participate in the group. In an ideal situation, there should be one practitioner for every three participants. Including successful graduates of past programs can also facilitate group work. Audiology students can also benefit from participating in group programs. The practicum helps reinforce both the theory discussed and the relevance of subjects taught in the classroom. The experience also provides an excellent opportunity to interact with a variety of older adults (Lesner, 1992).

BEGINNING THE GROUP

Beginnings can be stressful for all participants. The group leader and staff can use behaviors and gestures that help members feel at ease. Signs should be used to direct participants to the meeting room. A greeter should welcome the people to the session. Name tags should be provided to all participants with the names printed clearly and in large lettering.

The leader and staff should circulate and mingle with the participants before the session begins. The book *How to Work a Room: A Guide to Successfully Managing the Mingling* by Roane (1988) is highly recommended. Suggestions concerning a variety of topics, such as how to shake hands and maintain eye contact and the appropriate mind set (that you are the host rather than the guest), can facilitate mingling and ultimately set the appropriate psychosocial tone for the group sessions. Circulating among members at the beginning provides an opportunity to identify people who have severe communication difficulties. Once identified the leader should arrange for preferential seating or ALDs for those who need them.

Group members, including patients and professional staff, must be introduced. The group leader should begin and provide a model for other members to follow. Information about the type of hearing problems being experienced should be provided by the patients, and information about the backgrounds and interests of the professional staff should be provided. Older adults may question the skills of younger professionals, especially student clinicians, so it is important during the introductions to briefly describe the qualifications of the staff. In addition, providing a brief glimpse of participants' personal life contributes to an atmosphere of acceptance and facilitates the development of group cohesion.

The group leader should describe the purpose and goals of the sessions as clearly as possible. Meeting times and dates should be clarified. Requirements of group members and any related costs should be specified at the beginning.

MEETING CONTENT

Although sessions are outlined and have specific content (Appendix 9–1), it is important to maintain a flexible and relaxed approach. One need not become a slave to the agenda. The leader should address and react to member's questions, comments, and concerns. Participants should be encouraged to take notes.

At the beginning of each session, the leader briefly summarizes past meetings. (The session is also briefly summarized at the end.) This summary clarifies and highlights important points for the participants. It also tends to bring any participants who missed sessions up-to-date.

Hodgson (1994) suggested that three key words be kept in mind when presenting information—simplicity, redundancy, and feedback. Audiologic jargon should be avoided, and clear terminology and explanations accompanied by examples should be provided. Clarity and simplicity should not, however, result in talking down to the participants. Handouts and visual aids are useful as teaching tools.

In addition to the group work, it is important to provide individualized attention. If sufficient professional staff are involved, or if the number of participants is low, the individualized work can be provided either at the beginning or the end of the sessions. If this is not possible, individual sessions can be scheduled at other times.

The professional staff should maintain a sense of humor and persuade participants of the value of humor, mirth, and laughter. Because people with hearing impairments will continue to misperceive messages, having a sense of humor can lessen stress and strain. Humor has been found to be a coping mechanism for older adults (Vaillant, 1977). In addition, humor causes beneficial physiologic changes in older adults, including an improvement in alertness and memory (Fry, 1986).

EVALUATIONS OF THE GROUP

Evaluating the efficacy of group rehabilitation is difficult. Typical approaches to evaluation include experimental designs, quasiexperimental designs, or patient satisfaction surveys. Experimental designs require the use of a control group and are the most stringent approach. Quasiexperimental designs require a comparison group, but it is usually not possible to eliminate all alternative explanations for any given finding. Although satisfaction surveys are the least objective approach, they often yield valuable information for the practitioner (Barusch, 1991).

Patient satisfaction surveys can be easily developed for use with groups. Surveys provide qualitative data, but demand characteristics (Barusch, 1991) should be minimized. A demand characteristic is a tendency to imply or tell people what you want them to tell you. Demand characteristics can be minimized by having someone who did not participate in the training perform the evaluation and by assuring that the forms used do not identify the participant. Bias should be avoided in the wording of questions so that responses are not slanted. If questionnaires are used, they should assess participants' general responses to the program, their impressions about how the program has or has not affected their behavior, and which program elements were and were not particularly useful.

Binnie and Hession (1988) suggested that the success of a program can be defined by the attendance record of the participants, observations by the professional staff that participants are using effective communication strategies, or the use of self-report questionnaires to assess communication benefit. See Chapter 2 for a more thorough treatment of self-report questionnaires.

THE HEARING-AID ORIENTATION PROGRAM: A MODEL GROUP HEARING-CARE PROGRAM

The hearing-aid orientation program (HOP) is designed for use in a variety of clinical or community settings. Considering the number of clients who are newly fit with hearing instruments but stop wearing them, all people with hearing impairments are considered candidates for group membership, even those who do not have hearing instruments. The sessions are open and offered in 2-hour weekly sessions, and the sequence is repeated so that any missed sessions can be attended during subsequent series. The general goals of the HOP are to facilitate the patient's adjustment to amplification, to foster realistic expectations of hearing-aid use in people with hearing impairments and their significant others, and to maximize the patient's communication performance. In addition, emotional support is provided, and any particular problems being experienced by group participants are addressed.

A total of five sessions are offered and different topics are covered during each session. Appendix 9–1 lists group and individual activities included in the sessions. Although the outline includes suggested topics, it is important to maintain flexibility. Not all topics may be covered, some topics may be emphasized, or other topics of interest to group members may be added. When information is provided in response to questions from participants instead of in strictly lecture format, participation is maximized and the participants feel a greater sense of involvement. The emphasis of the sessions can be focused on the interest areas of the group. Interaction and group participation should be encouraged.

Session 1: Hearing Aids and Their Function

The purpose of the first session is to introduce and orient the group members to the program. The main topics of discussion are hearing aids and their function. Instruction in the use and care of hearing instruments and counseling to instill realistic expectations about the limitations and benefits are provided. Materials produced by Wayner (1990a,b) are suited to this session. Hearing-aid adjustments are made during the first session. The ability of participants to insert, remove, and use the controls of their hearing aids is assessed. Practice time is provided.

Session 2: Hearing and Hearing Loss

The focus of the second session is on hearing and hearing loss. Sufficient time is not usually present during an audiological assessment to explain the nature and consequences of a person's hearing loss. Some audiologists insist on explaining results with the use of the audiogram, not realizing the esoteric nature of the terms and symbols used. The HOP provides an opportunity to explain the patient's audiogram. During the second session the function of the ear, audiometric testing and results, and the effect of the hearing loss, especially in terms of speech perception, are examined. Individual sessions can be used to further explain the nature of the participant's hearing loss, the effect of the loss, and the prognosis. If needed, further practice in handling the hearing aids can be provided.

Session 3: Assistive Technologies

The third session highlights ALDs. Marketing of ALDs, which tend to be high-technology items, requires, in the words of Naisbitt (1982), high touch. It is not enough to explain the devices and how they function; the devices must be demonstrated. It is even more effective if people with hearing impairments can try the devices in their homes. Demonstration units and loaners should be available. If home use is not possible, demonstrating ALDs in a home-like atmosphere such as that described by Binnie and Hession (1988) is desirable. For people with severe listening problems, a home visit to demonstrate ALDs can be particularly productive. During the visit, the audiologist can assess the particular problems that exist in the home and ideally install trial devices.

One caution is that it is possible to overwhelm participants with a tabletop full of wires and gizmos. It is best to group the ALDs (signaling, telephone, group) or to demonstrate only units that appear to be appropriate if a home-like demonstration room or display is not available. Information about the availability of the devices in the community should be provided and the effects of the Americans with Disabilities Act should be discussed.

Session 4: Auditory and Visual Nature of Speech

It is a rare person who has contemplated the acoustic and visual nature of speech. So speech acoustics, the effects of noise and reverberation, and the visual perception of speech are discussed in the fourth session. Particular emphasis is given to the effect of hearing loss on speech perception. The use of an audiogram on which familiar sounds are listed at their approximate frequency and intensity is a valuable teaching tool.

The benefits of combined audiovisual perception are emphasized and demonstrated. It is stressed that the use of combined auditory and visual input optimizes speech perception for both people with hearing impairments and people with normal hearing (Massaro, 1987). Because there is a widespread notion, encouraged by spy movies, that it is possible to speechread everything, even in the dark and at a distance of several miles, the limitations of speechreading are discussed (Jeffers & Barley, 1971). Group speechreading tasks, during which the factors that contribute to success are highlighted, provide practice and demonstration of important speechreading principles. Use of the board game *Read My Lips*, manufactured by Pressman (Pressman Toy Corp., New Brunswick, NJ 08901) and available in toy stores, is an enjoyable way to provide speechreading opportunities.

Demonstrations of the benefits of audiovisual speech perception can be provided with the use of video-taped speech. Participants should first be instructed to speechread the visual portion of the tape with no audio. Then, only the auditory signal should be provided, but at a poor S/N. The reduction in S/N can be accomplished either by reducing the volume of the video monitor or by introducing noise. Participants should then be asked to listen and determine what was said when only the audio portion is played. Finally, with the S/N set to the same setting at which participants were having difficulty, they are asked to watch and listen. The improvement in ease of perception is quite obvious.

The detrimental effect of noise on speech perception is emphasized. Participants are questioned concerning listening situations that provide them with the greatest difficulty. Potential solutions to the problems are then explored by the group.

Considering the high prevalence of visual problems among older adults (see Chapter 1) and the need to maximize visual input, an important component of the fourth session is the administration of a visual screening. It is not uncommon for audiologists, who are sometimes so focused on the sense of hearing that they forget about the other senses, to provide speechreading training or audiovisual integration training to people who are functionally blind. Visual screenings can be easily provided with devices such as the Titmus Vision Tester (Titmus-Titmus Optical Co., Inc., Petersburg, VA), the Orthorater (Orthorater-Stereooptical, Chicago, IL), or a standard Snellen chart.

Session 5: Communication Strategies

The goal of the final session is to teach people with hearing impairments and their significant others how to engineer the acoustic, visual, and psychosocial environments to optimize communication and safety. In addition, various strategies, including anticipatory and repair strategies, designed to maximize communication are introduced for both people with hearing impairments and their significant others. Practice time and role-playing are provided. The materials prepared by Kaplan et al (1987) and Erber (1988; 1993) are highly recommended for use during this session.

The differences between assertiveness, aggression, and passivity are discussed. Role-playing or video tapes are used to demonstrate effective and noneffective behaviors (Trychin, 1987).

Final assessments and recommendations should be made. Participants are invited to return, and they are encouraged to bring or refer friends. In fact, successful graduates of HOPs make excellent participants and have reported that they have benefited from repeat attendance. Diplomas made with generally available software (Miller, 1990) are presented to each participant.

REFERENCES

Bally, S.J., & Kaplan, H. (1988). The Gallaudet University aural rehabilitation elderhostels. *Journal of the Academy of Rehabilitative Audiology, 21,* 99–112.

Barr, J. (1988). Group treatment: The logical choice. In B.B. Shadden (Ed.), *Communication behavior and aging: A source book for clinicians* (pp. 329–340). Baltimore: Williams & Wilkins.

Barusch, A.S. (1991). *Elder care: Family training and support.* Newbury Park: Sage.

Binnie, C., & Hession, C. (1988). *Communication training program for hearing-impaired adults: Accountability and marketability.* Presented at the Annual Meeting of the American Speech-Language-Hearing Association, November 18-21, 1988, Boston.

Brammer, L.M. (1981). What is a helping relationship? In J. E. Myers (Ed.), *Counseling older persons. Volume III. A trainer's manual for basic helping skills* (pp. 103–110). Falls Church: American Personnel and Guidance Association.

Brooks, D.N., (1979). Counseling and its effect on hearing aid use. *Scandinavian Audiology, 8,* 101–107.

Brooks, D.N. (1985). Factors relating to under-use of hearing aids. *British Journal of Audiology, 19,* 211–217.

Clark, J.G. (1994). Understanding, building, and maintaining relationships with patients. In J.G. Clark & F.N. Martin (Eds.), *Effective counseling in audiology: Perspectives and practice* (pp. 18–37). Englewood Cliffs: Prentice-Hall.

Corey, G., & Corey, M.S. (1977). *Groups: Process and practice.* Monterey: Brooks/Cole.

Erber, N.P. (1988). *Communication therapy for hearing-impaired adults.* Abbotsford: Clavis.

Erber, N.P. (1993). *Communication and adult hearing loss.* Abbotsford: Clavis.

Fisher, P.K., & Games, D.C. (1993). Finding funding for clients with special needs. *Hearsay, 8,* 38–39.

Fry, W.F. (1986). Humor, physiology, and the aging process. In L. Nahemow, K.A. McCluskey-Fawcett, & P.E. McGhee (Eds.), *Humor and aging* (pp. 81–98). Orlando: Academic Press.

Hardick, E.J., & Lesner, S.A. (1979). The need for audiologic habilitation: A different perspective. *Journal of the Academy of Rehabilitative Audiology, 12,* 21–29.

Hiatt L.G. (1990). Environmental factors in rehabilitation of disabled elderly people. In S.J. Brody & L.G. Pawlson (Eds.), *Aging and rehabilitation: The state of the practice* (pp. 150–164). New York: Springer Publishing.

Hickson, L., Hamilton, L., & Orange, S.P. (1986). Factors associated with hearing aid use. *Australian Journal of Audiology, 8,* 37–41.

Hodgson, W.R. (1994). Audiologic counseling. In J. Katz (Ed.), *Handbook of clinical audiology* (4th ed.) (pp. 616–623). Baltimore: Williams & Wilkins.

Jeffers, J., & Barley, M. (1971). *Speechreading (lipreading).* Springfield: Thomas.

Kaplan, H., Bally, S.J., & Garretson, C. (1987). *Speechreading: A way to improve understanding.* Washington: Gallaudet University Press.

Kapteyn, T.S. (1977). Satisfaction with fitted hearing aids. *Scandinavian Audiology, 6,* 147–156.

Kemp, B. (1990). The psychosocial context of geriatric rehabilitation. In B. Kemp, K. Brummel-Smith, & J.W. Ramsdell (Eds.), *Geriatric rehabilitation* (pp. 41–57). Boston: Little, Brown.

Lesner, S.A. (1992). Audiologic rehabilitation for older adults: Who needs it more, students or clients? *Hearsay, 7,* 25–29.

Massaro, D. (1987). *Speech perception by ear and eye: A paradigm for psychological inquiry.* Hillsdale: Lawrence Erlbaum.

Miller, G.C. (1990). *Laser award maker* (computer program). Grand Rapids: Baudville.

Montgomery, A.A. (1991). Aural rehabilitation: Review and preview. In G. Studebaker, F. Bess, & L. Beck (Eds.), *The Vanderbilt hearing aid report II* (pp. 223–231). Parkton: York.

Naisbitt, J. (1982). *Megatrends: Ten new directions transforming our lives.* New York: Warner.

Roane, S. (1988). *How to work a room: A guide to successfully managing the mingling.* New York: Sapolsky.

Roberts, S.D., & Bouchard, K.R. (1989). Establishing rapport in rehabilitative audiology. *Journal of the Academy of Rehabilitative Audiology, 22,* 67–73.

Rose, S.D. (1989) Preparing for group therapy: Planning treatment and orienting members. In S.D. Rose (Ed.), *Working with adults in groups: Integrating cognitive-behavioral and small group strategies* (pp. 45–71). San Francisco: Jossey-Bass.

Ross, M. (1987). Aural rehabilitation revisited. *Journal of the Academy of Rehabilitative Audiology, 20,* 13–23.

Rubinstein, A., & Cherry, R. (1988). The effect of letters on requests for clinic services following hearing aid prescription. *Journal of the Academy of Rehabilitative Audiology, 21,* 121–128.

Surr, R.K., Schuchman, G.I., & Montgomery, A.A. (1978). Factors influencing use of hearing aids. *Archives of Otolaryngology, 104,* 732–736.

Toseland, R.W. (1990). *Group work with older adults.* New York: New York University Press.

Trychin, S. (1987). *Communication rules for hard of hearing people* (videotape). Washington: Gallaudet University Press.

Vaillant, G.E. (1977). *Adaptation to life.* Boston: Little, Brown.

Vash, C. (1981). *The psychology of disability.* New York: Springer Publishing.

Ward, P.R., & Gowers, J.L. (1980). Fitting hearing aids: The effects of method of instruction. *British Journal of Audiology, 14,* 15–18.

Wayner, D.S. (1990a). *The hearing aid handbook: Clinician's guide to client orientation.* Washington: Gallaudet University Press.

Wayner, D.S. (1990b). *The hearing aid handbook: User's guide for adults.* Washington: Gallaudet University Press.

Appendix 9–1

Hearing Aid Orientation Program (HOP)

SESSION 1: HEARING AIDS AND THEIR FUNCTION

Group Topics

A. Introduction of professional staff and participants
   1. Professional staff
      a. Name
      b. Position
      c. Background experience
      d. Professional interests
   2. Participants
      a. Name
      b. Where they are from
      c. Type of hearing problems
      d. Interesting facts about self
B. General review of program goals, procedures, activities.
C. General introduction to hearing aids
   1. Basic operation (miniature public address system)
   2. Benefits
   3. Limitations
      a. Cannot differentiate between speech and noise
      b. Distortion introduced by the hearing loss will remain
   4. Hearing-aid fitting procedures
D. Controls, parts, and functions of hearing aids
   1. M-T-O switch
   2. Volume control
   3. Battery compartment
   4. Microphone opening
   5. Receiver opening
   6. Earmold
   7. Vents
   8. Tubing

E. Batteries
    1. Types and sizes
    2. Battery life
    3. Storage of batteries
    4. Costs and suggestions about where to purchase batteries
    5. Battery testers
    6. Accidental swallowing of batteries
        a. Battery ingestion hotline (202-625-3333)
        b. Tamper-proof battery compartments
F. Care of hearing aids
    1. How to clean the hearing aid and earmold
    2. Wax removal tools and their use
    3. Dehumidifiers, dry aid kits, and forced-air blowers
    4. How to store the hearing aid when it is not being used
    5. Situations to avoid: extremes of heat, humidity
    6. Pets and hearing aids
G. Hearing-aid warranty information
H. Hearing-aid insurance
I. General trouble-shooting information
    1. Causes and prevention of feedback
    2. Problems related to batteries
    3. Problems related to cerumen and moisture

Group Counseling Topics

A. Group conversation to introduce members
B. Conversation about the following question: Have you been disappointed with your hearing aid?

Individual Counseling or Testing

A. Discuss and assess difficulties that patient identifies as most important
B. Determine that patient can handle the hearing aids, including insertion of the hearing aid and battery, and that patient can successfully manipulate the controls

SESSION 2: HEARING AND HEARING LOSS

Group Topics

A. Anatomy of the ear
B. Physiology of the ear

C. Common disorders of the ear (emphasis on problems experienced by group members)
   1. Impacted cerumen
   2. External otitis
   3. Perforated ear drums
   4. Negative middle ear pressure
   5. Otitis media
   6. Otosclerosis
   7. Negative pressure
   8. Drug-induced cochlear hearing losses
   9. Meniere syndrome
   10. Disease-induced cochlear hearing loss
   11. Vascular cochlear hearing loss
   12. Noise-induced hearing loss
   13. Age-related hearing loss
   14. Hearing loss due to the presence of tumors
   15. Tinnitus
   16. Other pathologic conditions of interest to the group

D. Types of hearing loss (site-of-lesion) and general consequences
   1. Conductive
      a. Attenuation of sounds
   2. Sensorineural
      a. Attenuation of sounds
      b. Distortion of sounds
   3. Mixed
      a. Attenuation of sounds
      b. Distortion of sounds
   4. Central—processing difficulty

E. How hearing losses are treated

F. Interpretation of an audiogram (including familiar sounds audiogram)
   1. Decibels
   2. Hertz
   3. Audiometric symbols
   4. Degrees of hearing loss
   5. Configuration of hearing losses

G. The audiologic test battery and its purpose
   1. Pure-tone thresholds
   2. Speech discrimination testing
   3. Immittance testing

H. Qualifications, training, and the role of various hearing-care professionals
   1. Audiologists
   2. Otolaryngologists
   3. Hearing-aid dispensers

Group Counseling Topics

A. Explanation of each patient's audiogram
B. Discussion of familiar sounds audiogram and patients' experiences
C. Demonstration tape of filtered speech for significant other
D. Further discussion concerning pathologic conditions of interest to the group

Individual Counseling or Testing

A. Further explanation of patient's audiometric results, if needed
B. Handicap profiles
C. Patient training in manipulation of hearing aid, if needed

SESSION 3: ASSISTIVE TECHNOLOGY

Group Topics

A. Situational limitations of hearing aids
   1. Noise
   2. Distance listening
   3. Signal-to-noise ratio
   4. Reverberation
B. Rationale and explanation of ALDs
C. Types of assistive listening device technologies
   1. Hard-wired systems
   2. Loop systems
   3. FM systems
   4. Infrared systems
D. Demonstration of assistive devices, including discussion of advantages, disadvantages and costs
   1. Large-area systems
   2. Interpersonal communication devices
   3. Telephone devices
   4. Television and radio devices
   5. Alerting devices
E. How to obtain or order assistive devices
F. Availability of ALDs in the community
G. The implications of the Americans with Disabilities Act

Individual Counseling or Testing

A. Listening questionnaire (see Chapter 6)
B. Recommendations about purchase or trial use of assistive technology
C. Practice with the use of devices
D. Practice with the use of hearing-aid telephone coils for those who have them

SESSION 4: AUDITORY AND VISUAL NATURE OF SPEECH

Group Topics

A. Speech acoustics
B. Effects of noise on speech perception (video tape demonstration)
C. Definition, demonstration, and discussion of the effect of reverberation on speech perception
D. Visible aspects of speech perception
E. Limitations of speechreading
    1. Low visibility of speech sounds
    2. Homophenous sounds (sounds that look alike)
    3. Speaker differences in speech sound production
    4. Rapidity of speech compared with ability of the eyes to follow
    5. Coarticulation effects
    6. Environmental restraints (eg, lighting, angle)
F. Advantages of audiovisual perception of speech (video tape demonstration)
G. Suggestions to optimize speechreading performance
H. Listening versus hearing

Group Activities

A. Visual, auditory, audiovisual tests of speech perception
B. Group-administered speechreading tests using speakers who vary in their visual intelligibility

Individual Counseling or Testing

Visual screening

SESSION 5: COMMUNICATION STRATEGIES

Group Topics

A. Need for and suggestions for manipulating acoustic, visual, and psychosocial environments
B. Assertiveness training
C. Coping strategies
    1. Anticipatory strategies
    2. Repair strategies
D. Suggestions for significant others to improve communication
E. Stress management
F. Advocacy
G. Self Help for Hard of Hearing People (SHHH)
H. Need for a sense of humor

Group Counseling and Discussion

A. How do group members contribute to their own communication problems?
B. Group members' suggestions for tips on communicating more effectively
C. Final questions and comments

Individual Counseling or Testing

A. Follow-up testing with handicap inventories or profiles
B. HOP satisfaction questionnaire
C. Final recommendations

Graduation

Chapter 10

Service Delivery Models for Older Adults with Hearing Impairments: Individual Sessions

Mary Beth Jennings

For practitioners who provide individual audiologic rehabilitation to older adults with hearing impairments, preparation time is premium. The purpose of this chapter is to provide practitioners with a practical outline of audiologic rehabilitation activities for their patients. Twenty-four individual sessions are provided. These sessions focus on speechreading training, auditory training, and conversational fluency. The sessions are presented in approximate order of increasing difficulty. The practitioner is encouraged to be creative and to refine each session to meet the client's abilities, potentials, and needs.

The sessions provide training of auditory (A), visual (V), and auditory-visual (AV) skills. They provide training at various levels of these skills, including detection, discrimination, identification, recognition, and comprehension. The sessions also provide training at various levels of linguistic skill. These levels include pragmatics, syntax, and semantics, similar to exercises outlined by Walther (1982) and Erber (1988). Training is also provided in the use of situational context to enhance the reception of the spoken message. These exercises are modeled after exercises by Erber (1988) and Jeffers and Barley (1979).

Practice is provided with environmental sounds (Haug & Haug, 1977; Windle & Stout, 1992); rhythm (Windle & Stout, 1992); intonation and stress (Mecklenburg et al, 1987); syllables, words, phrases, sentences, paragraphs, and stories (Jeffers & Barley, 1979; Jennings et al, 1991); and continuous discourse (De Filippo, 1988; Erber, 1988; Pichora-Fuller & Robertson, 1993). Although the use of background noise is not introduced until Session 17, it can be introduced earlier or later. The type and level of background noise can be varied at the practitioner's discretion. The goal is to provide a realistic noise background, one that challenges the patient without undesired frustration.

The practitioner is referred to other chapters in this book for a discussion of therapy goals, evaluation before intervention, and considerations in the remediation process.

SESSION ONE

1. The goals for therapy are discussed with the client. The client is asked to list his or her goals. The practitioner also lists his or her goals. The roles and responsibilities of the practitioner and of the client are discussed.

2. The term of therapy is discussed, and a contract is drawn up that outlines the number of sessions agreed upon, length and frequency of the sessions, and criteria for renewal of the contract after the initial contract has been fulfilled.

3. The practitioner encourages the involvement of significant others in the sessions and discusses their responsibilities within the sessions and in carryover.

4. The practitioner makes the client and significant others aware of other services available to them, such as counseling, vocational rehabilitation, employment services, assistive devices, and self-help groups. The practitioner also discusses possible sources of financial assistance and speech-language pathology, as necessary.

5. The topic of speechreading is introduced to the client. Speechreading the consonant sounds of English is reviewed with the client and handouts are provided. The sounds are as follows.

    Sounds that are very easy to speechread are made at the front of the mouth. The sounds "p", "b", and "m" are all made the same way on the lips. The lips come together and are then released. Examples of words with these sounds at the beginning are *pie, by,* and *my.* The sounds "r" and "w" are made in the same way on the lips. The lips are protruded with a narrow, rounded opening. For the "r", the tongue is at the top of the mouth, and the sides of the tongue are against the side teeth. Examples of words with these sounds at the beginning are *ring* and *wing.* The sounds "f" and "v" are made in the same way on the lips. The lower lip is brought into light contact with the upper teeth. Examples of words with these sounds at the beginning are *feel* and *veal.* The sound "th" is made by having the tongue protrude slightly between the teeth. Examples of words with "th" at the beginning are *this* and *though.*

    Sounds that are easy to speechread are made at the front of the mouth. The sounds "sh", "ch", and "j" are all made the same way on the lips. The lips are rounded and protruded. The tongue is near the top of the mouth. Examples of words with these sounds at the beginning are *shock, chalk,* and *jock.*

    Sounds that are difficult to speechread are made behind the front teeth and in the middle of the mouth. The sounds "t", "d", "n", "l", and "y" are all made the same way on the lips. The lips are in a relaxed position, and the tip of the tongue is behind the front teeth.

For "y", the sides of the tongue touch the insides of the teeth. Examples of words with these sounds at the beginning are *Tess*, *desk*, *Ness*, *less*, and *yes*. The sounds "s" and "z" are made in the same way on the lips. The lips are slightly spread, and the teeth are together. The tongue is at the top of the mouth. Examples of words with these sounds at the beginning are *sip* and *zip*.

Sounds that are very difficult to speechread are made in the back of the mouth. The sounds "k" and "g" are made in the same way on the lips. The lips are open and are in a relaxed position. The back of the tongue is at the top of the mouth. Examples of words with these sounds at the beginning are *came* and *game*. The sound /h/ is made with the mouth in a relaxed position. There are no visible movements. Examples of words made with this sound at the beginning are *hello* and *how*.

6. The practitioner presents words from each viseme group, V-only, A-only, and AV and has the client identify from which viseme group the beginning sound belongs.

7. The practitioner asks the client to practice and learn the viseme groups at home with his or her significant others.

SESSION TWO

1. The viseme groups are reviewed with the client to ensure familiarity with the consonant sounds of English.

2. Factors that affect communication for people who are hard-of-hearing are discussed. The client's experiences related to these factors and solutions to difficulties are discussed. Some of the factors that affect communication for people with hearing impairments include visual and auditory difficulties. Examples are as follows:

   a. Poor lighting that casts shadows on speakers' faces or shines into a listener's eyes makes it difficult to speechread.

   b. Visual distractions and background noise make it difficult to concentrate on and hear the speaker.

   c. The greater the distance from the speaker, the more difficult it is to see the speaker's face for speechreading. It is also more difficult to hear the speaker from a distance.

   d. Objects that cover the speaker's face or distortion caused by chewing make it difficult to hear and speechread the speaker.

   e. Listening to a speaker over a public address system, radio, or television can be more difficult than listening to a speaker one-on-one, live-voice.

    f.   Poor visual acuity makes speechreading difficult. Good visual acuity is necessary for successful speechreading.

3.   Initial consonant identification exercise. A list of 20 groupings of sounds are given to the client. The practitioner presents one sound in the grouping to the client. The client must identify which sound was presented. Items from the groupings are presented in V-only, A-only, and AV conditions.

ba sa ra	na sa wa	ra ba na
pa fa ga	la ha tha	wa cha ta
ma cha ta	ya ba sha	ka za fa
fa wa tha	sha da za	ga pa sha
va ma ella	cha ka ya	
tha na ka	ja ra ga	
ta za va	sa ha va	
da pa ja	za ma da	

4.   Medial consonant identification exercise. A list of 20 groupings are given to the client. The practitioner presents one sound in the grouping to the client. The client identifies which sound was presented. Items from the groupings are presented in V-only, A-only, and AV conditions.

aba asa ara	aya aba asha
apa afa aga	asha ada aza
ama acha ata	acha aka aya
afa awa atha	aja ara aga
ava ama ala	asa aha ava
ata aza ava	ara aba ana
ada apa aja	awa acha ata
ana asa awa	aka aza afa
ala aha atha	aga apa asha

5.   Final consonant identification exercise. A list of 20 groupings is given to the client. The practitioner presents one sound in the grouping to the client. The client identifies which sound was presented. Items from the groupings are presented in V-only, A-only, and AV conditions.

ab as ak	ash ad az
ap af ag	ach ak at
am ach at	aj ag az
af al ad	as av ag
av am al	am az ad
ath an ak	ak az af
at az av	ag ap ash
ad ap aj	ag ab az
al ap ag	an as ap
ath as ak	as ath ab

6. Homophenous word exercise. The client is given the following list of words. For each word, the client is asked to identify other words that would look the same on the lips.

   pan
   feel
   too
   ship
   sink
   rip
   coal

7. The following homophenous words are presented to the client V-only, A-only, and AV. Each word is presented in a sentence, and the client is asked to identify which word was used. The sentences are first presented V-only, then A-only, and finally in the AV condition.

   a. pan   She saw the flames from the fire in the pan.
      ban   She couldn't find the book and then remembered the ban.
      man   She remembered his name and knew about the man.
   b. feel   He wanted to feel the material.
      veal   He had veal for dinner.
   c. Tess   My sister's name is Tess.
      desk   My office has a desk.
      Ness   My brother saw Loch Ness.
      less   My weight was much less.
      yes   My mother would say yes.
   d. ship   They sailed in a ship.
      chip   The mug had a chip.
   e. sink   There were dishes in the sink.
      zinc   The stone contained some zinc.
   f. rip   She had a rip in her shirt.
      whip   She had to whip the cream.
   g. coal   The coal was very black.
      goal   The goal was almost met.
      hole   The hole was pretty big.

8. The client is asked to compile a diary and analyze communication situations that are difficult and to bring the diary and the analysis.

SESSION THREE

1. The practitioner and the client review the diary of difficult listening situations and discuss how to make these situations easier for communication.

2. The topic of factors that influence success in communication is introduced. Factors that influence success in communication include the persons's physical state, analytic skills, attitude, and the situation itself.

a.   The client's physical state can influence the ability to concentrate on the speaker. If the client is tired or unwell, it may be difficult for them to concentrate on the speaker and therefore communication is more difficult.

b.   Clients' analytic skills can influence their ability to analyze the situation when communication breaks down, to identify what caused the problem, and to help solve the problem.

c.   The client's attitude can influence success in communication. Having a positive attitude and an acceptance of the hearing loss can help the client cope better with communication. The client is reminded that even in life in general, attitude is 99 percent.

d.   The situation itself can influence success in communication; some situations may be easier than others for communication. There may be greater success in communication in situations that are not stressful and involve others with whom the client feels comfortable.

2.   Exercise in the identification of environmental sounds. The exercise is presented A-only and AV using pictures of the sources of the environmental sounds. The purpose of the exercise is to have the client identify sounds in the environment while using amplification. The client listens to an audio tape of environmental sounds, such as a vacuum cleaner, kettle whistling, dog barking, fire engine siren, water running, and music on the radio, and is asked to identify the sound. This activity can be particularly helpful for new users of hearing aids.

3.   Exercise in the recognition of rhythm. The purpose of the exercise is to have the client become aware of the rhythm of speech. The exercise is presented V-only, A-only, and AV. The client is instructed to tap the number of syllables in the following words. The words are presented AV the first time, A-only the second time, and V-only the third time.

dime	follow	parliament	foe	visit	manager
vine	baby	furniture	theme	poppy	verify
toad	memo	luckily	ring	yellow	charity
home	cherry	carefully	ball	woody	basketball
pop	nasty	hospital	mall	restful	thoughtfulness
sue	hobby	yesterday	wig	thankful	shakily
none	timid	rarity	lip	dopey	granary
yes	likely	tamarack	shoe	showy	diligent
chip	joker	neutralize	jam	sorry	jauntily
call	carry	situate	go	given	warily

4.   Exercise in the recognition of rhythm in sentences. The client is asked to tap the number of syllables in the following sentences. The sentences are presented AV the first time, A-only the second time, and V-only the third time.

The grapes grew on a vine.
He likes to play baseball.
Strawberry jam tastes good on bread.
I didn't see anything.
She went home after work.
The heel broke off the shoe.
I visited them last week.
They have a new baby.
Did you get my memo?
That's nothing new.
We had cherry pie for dessert.
I was only joking.
The manager was out.
The basketball game is at two o'clock.
Her mother is in the hospital.
I saw him yesterday.
He is a diligent worker.
Their dog is very timid.
I was thankful for the help.
I'm very sorry.

5. Exercise in the recognition of rhythm in a poem. The client is asked to listen to the poem when it is presented AV. The poem is then presented A-only and the client is asked to tap the rhythm of the poem line by line.

   The north wind did blow,
   Over the snow,
   But spring was nowhere to be found.
   There was not a sound,
   Over the ground,
   But the sun smiled and spring saw that glow.

6. Tracking exercise. The client is instructed to repeat verbatim what is said. If the client is unable to repeat some or all of the words, he or she is instructed to ask for clarification from the speaker using the following rank-ordered strategies. First, the client asks the speaker to repeat the segment that was missed. Second, the client asks the speaker to rephrase the segment that was missed. Third, the client can ask a question that might help fill-in the missing information. Finally, the client can ask for the topic or key word. If the client is unaware that some of the information has been misinterpreted or missed, the speaker repeats the missed information.

The practitioner provides a copy of the poem used for the rhythm exercise for the client to follow. The client is asked to read the poem and then track the poem one line at a time. The tracking is first done in the AV condition then repeated in the A-only and V-only conditions.

7. The client is asked to practice tapping the rhythm of poems at home V-only, A-only, and AV with significant others.

SESSION FOUR

1. Communication strategies. The following strategies for making communication easier are discussed with the client, and the client is asked to discuss his or her experiences.

Strategies for Making Communication Easier

   a. Have the speaker speak a little slower.

   b. Have the speaker speak in a slightly louder voice but not shout.

   c. Have the speaker face you when speaking.

   d. Have the speaker repeat what he or she said only once. After that, he or she tries to rephrase the utterance and use words that are easier to hear and speechread.

   e. Have the speaker tell you the topic or give you a key word.

   f. Have the speaker spell the missed word, key word, or topic.

   g. Have the speaker write down the message, if necessary.

   h. Always confirm that you received the correct message.

2. Exercise for identifying words that are given auditory emphasis in a sentence. Being able to identify words that are given auditory emphasis in a sentence can help the client identify words that are important to the meaning of the sentence. The practitioner explains that the client will hear each sentence three times. A list of the sentences, without the emphasized words identified, is read to the client. The client is asked to identify the word in the sentence that is given auditory emphasis. The sentence is presented A-only and then presented AV.

   a. His ignorance *can* be helped.
      His *ignorance* can be helped.
      His ignorance can be helped.

   b. *You* were planning to go.
      You *were* planning to go.
      You were *planning* to go.

   c. *What* was his name?
      What was *his* name?
      What *was* his name?

   d. No one *knows* her.
      No one knows her.
      No one knows *her*.

e. When *will* it open?
    When will *it* open?
    When will it open?
f. *He* knows the teacher.
    He *knows* the teacher.
    He knows the *teacher*.
g. I love *chocolate* cake.
    I *love* chocolate cake.
    I love chocolate cake.
h. The river was very *long*.
    The river was *very* long.
    The *river* was very long.
i. I *hope* you have a happy birthday.
    I hope *you* have a happy birthday.
    I hope you have a *happy* birthday.
j. Please *leave* by the exit.
    Please leave *by* the exit.
    Please leave by the exit.

3. Exercise for identifying intonation in the voice. Intonation is the rising or falling of intensity in the voice that tells the listener if the utterance is a question, statement, or a command. The practitioner explains that the client will hear each sentence three times. A list of the sentences is read to the client. The client is asked to identify whether the sentence is a statement, question, or command. The sentence is presented A-only and then AV.

> Don't tell my father.
> You must listen to me.
> She wears size eight shoes.
> Look for him at the corner.
> Show her the picture.
> I want a cup of coffee.
> You should read the newspaper.
> I will like this movie.
> Tell him to go away.
> Close the door.

4. Exercise for identifying the rate of speech. When a speaker speaks too quickly or too slowly, the utterance can be more difficult to understand. The practitioner explains that the client will hear a passage three times. The client is asked to identify whether the passage was read slowly, quickly, or moderately. The practitioner reads the passage three times. The first time the passage is read quickly. The second time the passage is read at a moderate pace. The third time the passage is read very slowly.

After the three readings, the client and practitioner discuss at which speed they found the paragraph to be most intelligible.

I just heard the weather forecast. Tomorrow it will be mainly cloudy with scattered snow flurries. The probability of precipitation is eighty percent and the high will be near five degrees.

5. Explain that the poem used for tracking in Session Three will be tracked again. The client is instructed to read the poem and then turn the page over. The poem is tracked one line at a time. The first time, the poem is tracked AV. The second time, the poem is tracked A-only. The third time, the poem is tracked V-only.

6. The client is asked to practice identifying intonation and emphasis with significant others. He or she is also asked to practice finding the best rate of speech for understanding with significant others.

SESSION FIVE

1. The topic of gestures and facial expressions is introduced. Gestures and facial expressions can provide valuable information regarding the meaning of an utterance and help the client confirm that he or she has received the correct message. The following are some gestures that could be used by the client and significant others to help with communication.

   a. A raised forefinger moved up in front of puckered lips means "quiet."
   b. A fist with an extended and bent forefinger moving back and forth means "come here."
   c. Both hands open outward with the palms up and making a few lifting movements means "speak louder."
   d. Both hands open palm down and making a few downward movements means "speak softer."
   e. Both hands brought together with the palms touching means "please."
   f. Nodding the head up and down means "yes."
   g. Shaking the head side to side means "no."

2. Exercise for discriminating word length. The client is instructed that two words will be presented. The client is asked to tell the practitioner whether the words are the same length (have the same number of syllables) or are different. Three lists are given. The first list is presented AV, the second list is presented A-only, and the third list is presented V-only.

List One	List Two	List Three
dime timid	follow furniture	chip dam
mall pop	home hospital	sorry yellow
yesterday yes	tamarack diligent	hobby given
rarity warily	restful woody	parliament manager
home jam	go uncanny	shakily jauntily
follow verify	thankfully thoughtfulness	visit foe
lip likely	granary yesterday	baby ball
theme thankful	cherry joker	neutralize none
sue shoe	nasty timid	situate sorry
memo poppy	wig ring	charity chip

3. Exercise for identifying word length. The client is given the preceding lists of words. One of the two words is presented, and the client is instructed to identify which of the two words was presented. The first list is presented AV, the second list A-only, and the third list V-only.

4. Exercise for discriminating the length of sentences. The client is instructed that two sentences will be presented. The client is asked to tell the practitioner whether the sentences are the same length (have the same number of syllables) or are different. The first list of sentences is presented AV, the second list A-only, and the third list V-only.

List One

a. I'm very sorry.
   He was timid.
b. Is this your shoe?
   She bought a ring.
c. Will you visit me?
   Did you ever go?
d. I like cherry jam.
   She ate apple pie.
e. Brush your teeth.
   Wash your face.
f. He is a diligent worker.
   I don't use furniture polish.
g. Don't throw out the wrapper.
   Did you see that movie?
h. The piano was tuned last week.
   One newspaper said it was true.
i. Shovel the walkway.
   Haven't you finished?
j. Black smoke filled the room.
   The car needs some gas.

List Two

a. Popcorn is my favorite snack food.
    Seafood is a wonderful fast meal.
b. They lived right around the corner.
    Phone me and repeat the story.
c. Go home.
    Who knows?
d. Be quiet.
    She listened.
e. He was timid.
    Is this your shoe?
f. She bought a ring.
    He is a diligent worker.
g. I don't use furniture polish.
    The piano was tuned last week.
h. Carry on.
    All right.
i. One newspaper said it was true.
    Who knows?
j. Be quiet.
    Will you visit me?

List Three

a. Go home.
    I'm very sorry.
b. Brush your teeth.
    Don't throw out the wrapper.
c. Did you ever go?
    Popcorn is my favorite snack food.
d. Did you see that movie?
    She listened.
e. Seafood is a wonderful fast meal.
    Wash your face.
f. Carry on.
    Black smoke filled the room.
g. Shovel the walkway.
    They lived right around the corner.
h. I like cherry jam.
    All right.
i. The car needs some gas.
    Haven't you finished?
j. Phone me and repeat the story.
    She ate apple pie.

5. Identification of sentence length. The client is given the preceding list of sentences. The client is instructed that two sentences will be presented.

The client is asked to identify which of the two sentences was presented. The first list is presented AV, the second list A-only, and the third list V-only.

6. Explain that the poem tracked in Session Three will be tracked again, this time without prior reading. First, the poem is tracked AV. The second time, the poem is tracked A-only, and the third time V-only.

7. The client is instructed to compile a dictionary of gestures that the client and his or her significant others agree to use to supplement communication.

SESSION SIX

1. The topic of how to get the most out of communication is introduced. To get the most out of communication, the client needs to use the following tools:

   a. Speechreading, which is the interpretation of lip movements and their associated sound groupings
   b. Gestures and facial expressions, which can enhance the meaning of the utterance
   c. Intonation, stress, and rhythm, that is, audible changes in the voice that provide emphasis, clues to word length, number of syllables, and voice patterns for questions, statements, and commands
   d. Knowledge of language, which helps people eliminate what does not make sense and helps fill in missing information
   e. Residual hearing, that is, use of hearing aids and assistive listening devices to optimize the auditory signal
   f. Contextual cues, that is, clues gained from knowledge of the topic, subject, or situation

2. Exercise for using context. The client is given a category and told he or she will be presented with members of the category and asked to identify those members. The first category is presented AV. The second category is presented A-only, and the third V-only.

Birds	Beverages	Trees
robin	coffee	oak
blue jay	tea	elm
cardinal	milk	spruce
finch	soda pop	pine
dove	water	birch
thrush	juice	mountain ash
turkey	cocoa	maple
nightingale	cider	willow
sparrow	lemonade	juniper
grosbeak	ale	larch

3. Exercise using association words. The client is presented with a series of written word lists with one word missing in each list. The missing words are presented, and the client is asked to identify them. Each missing word is first presented V-only. If the missing word is not identified, the list is presented A-only. If the word is still not identified, it is presented AV.

    a. cold, snow, ice, *freezing*
    b. rain, shower, sprinkle, *cloudburst*
    c. value, worth, appreciate, *treasure*
    d. zone, area, region, *realm*
    e. jam, preserve, raspberry, *marmalade*
    f. break, fracture, chip, *smash*
    g. nervous, flustered, tense, *worried*
    h. think, brainstorm, puzzle, *contemplate*

4. The client is presented with a situation AV. The client is then presented with an utterance that might be heard in that situation. The client is asked to repeat the utterance. First, the utterance is presented V-only. If the utterance cannot be repeated, it is presented A-only. Finally, the utterance is presented AV.

    a. Shopping for groceries: "Where can I find the bread?"
    b. At the post office in April: "Have you mailed in your income tax return yet?"
    c. Around the campfire: "Do you want to toast marshmallows?"
    d. At the beach, with a tube of suntan lotion in hand: "Would you like me to put lotion on your back?"
    e. Someone jumps into the swimming pool: "The water is freezing!"
    f. At the newsstand, pointing to the front page of a newspaper: "Did you see the headlines?"
    g. In a long line at the grocery store checkout: "Why don't they open another check-out?"
    h. While doing stacks of dishes: "It looks like we saved these up for a week!"
    i. In the car at a four-way stop: "Turn left here."
    j. Sitting in front of the television, looking through the program guide: "There's a good movie on at eight o'clock."

5. The client is presented AV with a name, place, or situation. A list of sentences related to the situation is presented, and the client is asked to repeat the sentences. The sentences are first presented V-only. If the sentence cannot be repeated, it is presented A-only, and if the sentence still cannot be repeated, it is presented AV.

Coffee Shop

> I'll have a large cup of coffee.
> Would you like anything to eat?
> Do you have jelly donuts?

I like cream and sugar in my coffee.
Do you have hot chocolate?
Can I have a toasted bagel with cream cheese?
Where is the non-smoking section?
Do you want to sit at the counter?
There's a booth available that seats four people.
I only have a fifteen minute break.

6. The poem tracked in Session Three is tracked again, this time without any written information. The client is asked the following questions about the poem after the tracking is completed:

In what season does the poem take place?
What season will follow?
What is covering the ground?
What was blowing? What was smiling?

SESSION SEVEN

1. Exercise for using context. The client is presented with members of a category, asked to repeat the members, and then guess the category. The first list of members is presented AV, the second A-only, and the third list V-only.

Animals	Fabrics	Houseplants
bear	cotton	dieffenbacchia
moose	wool	geranium
deer	polyester	African violet
beaver	gabardine	pothos
rabbit	nylon	spider plant
squirrel	silk	fern
ground hog	rayon	jade plant
woodchuck	acetate	kalanchoe
lynx	tulle	prayer plant
jaguar	satin	fittonia

2. The client is presented AV with a topic or situation and an utterance heard in that situation. A response to the utterance is presented to the client, and the client is asked to repeat the response. The first time the response is presented V-only. If the client cannot repeat the utterance, it is presented A-only. If the client still cannot repeat the utterance, it is presented AV.

    a. At a restaurant: "I love seafood." "I prefer prime rib."
    b. At a gas station: "The gas prices went up again." "How much is a gallon of gas?"
    c. Talking to a store clerk: "Do you carry white blouses?" "We have a few over on that rack."

242 Hearing Care for the Older Adult

    d. Watching television: "I can't miss the news." "What time does it begin?"

    e. Listening to the radio: "I love that song." "So do I."

    f. At the dinner table: "This meal is excellent." "Thank you!"

    g. Doing the laundry: "Should I wash my black shirt in hot water?" "No. You should use cold water."

    h. At the bank: "I need some more checks." "How many would you like?"

    i. At the grocery store: "Do you carry whole-wheat flour?" "No, we only have all-purpose flour."

    j. Talking to your grandchildren: "How was school today?" "There was a big fight at recess."

3. Exercise using common phrases. A word is presented AV to the client. A common phrase containing the word is presented. The client is asked to repeat the phrase. The phrases are first presented V-only. If the client cannot repeat the phrase, it is presented A-only. If the client still cannot repeat the phrase, it is presented AV.

    a. slow—as slow as molasses

    b. worth—not worth a dime

    c. fish—fish and chips

    d. cows—a herd of cows

    e. clothes—a change of clothes

    f. cold—as cold as ice

    g. hot—as hot as blazes

    h. weight—worth its weight

    i. storm—talk up a storm

    j. write—write a letter

4. The client is given a written list of sentences. The last word is missing from each sentence. The sentences, including the missing words, are presented V-only the first time. The client is asked to repeat the missing words. If the client cannot repeat the missing words, the sentence is repeated A-only. If the client still cannot repeat the missing words, the sentence is repeated AV.

Please close the *door.*
The sun was so bright I closed the *curtains.*
Turn left at the *corner.*
He spilled coffee on the *carpet.*
Listen to that loud *noise.*
Wipe the floor with a damp *mop.*
The ship was sailing on the *water.*
Please put out the *garbage.*
Use a hammer and a nail to fasten the *board.*
I've read that book *before.*

5. A story is presented. The first sentence is presented, and the sentences that follow are added one at a time until all of the sentences are presented in succession. The client is asked to repeat the sentences as presented by the practitioner. The sentences are first presented V-only, then A-only, and finally AV.

> We just bought a puppy.
> Our puppy is three months old.
> We bought the puppy from a breeder.
> The puppy is a Shetland Sheepdog.
> We named her Coffee.
> Coffee is housebroken.
> She likes to run and play in the yard.
> We hope that Coffee will be with us for a long time.

6. Tracking. The client is given the story to read and is asked to turn the page over after the first reading. The story is tracked, V-only, A-only, and AV.

> Last spring, a pedestrian bridge was built in our town. It was built across the river. The river runs through the town. I enjoy walking across the bridge. Canada geese nest on the shores of the river. You can see lots of geese when you walk over the bridge.

SESSION EIGHT

1. A topic or situation and an utterance heard in the situation are presented AV. The client is asked to predict an appropriate response to the utterance.
   a. Talking to your boss: "Have you thought about my request for a raise?"
   b. Talking to a neighbor: "Did you hear the sirens last night?"
   c. At the doctor's office: "Do you need my health insurance information?"
   d. At the dentist's office: "I don't like the taste of the fluoride."
   e. At the market: "The fruit looks so fresh!"
   f. At the video store: "I love this movie!"
   g. At breakfast: "I don't like pancakes."
   h. At the dry cleaners: "You shrunk my sweater!"
   i. On a bus: "Are we close to Hanover Street?"
   j. In the garden: "These snails are real pests!"
2. The client is presented with a sentence AV. One word in the sentence is presented V-only. The client is asked to guess the word by using the context of the sentence.
   a. They spend the winter in _____.
   b. The boy had a _____ hat.

    c. At the farm, there were six _____.

    d. The road was covered with _____.

    e. I voted for _____ in the last election.

    f. I own two pairs of warm _____.

    g. What was her _____ name?

    h. I take a _____ to work.

    i. That shirt is made of _____.

    j. Our dog likes to eat _____.

3. A short story is presented AV. The last sentence of the story is presented in print, with some of the words left out. The practitioner presents the words V-only, and the client is asked to fill in the missing words. If the words cannot be filled in, the sentence is presented A-only and then AV.

    a. My father and I went fishing. I put the worm on my hook and lowered the line into the water. After about ten minutes, I could feel something tugging at the line. I said: "I think I *caught* a *fish!*"

    b. Over a period of a year I had noticed my vision getting poorer. I made an appointment to have my eyes tested. At the end of the examination, I was told: "Your *vision* is *poor* and you need *glasses.*"

    c. I like to listen to music. I also tend to listen to music at a loud volume. One day, I had the music up so loud that my father said, "*Turn* that music *down!*"

    d. We have a big vegetable garden. We like to grow lots of tomatoes. Yesterday, we had about a dozen ripe tomatoes. When we went out to pick them this morning, they were gone. I said, "Who *stole* my *tomatoes?*"

    e. I have a long drive to work and back home each day. On my way home yesterday, I looked down at the fuel gauge. The gauge was registering empty. I thought, "I had better *get some gas.*"

    f. Our dog likes to roll in the mud. He went out after we had a rain storm and came home covered with dirt. I said, "You need *a bath.*"

    g. We had ten friends over for dinner last night. By the time they left, dishes were piled high in the kitchen. It was midnight when I said, "Let's leave *the dishes* until *morning.*"

    h. I was cleaning in the basement when the phone started to ring. I knew that my husband was upstairs so I yelled, "Please *answer* the *phone.*"

    i. Friends of ours dropped by last evening. We talked for a while and then I started to feel thirsty. I asked my guests. "Would you *like something* to *drink?*"

    j. We had a big snowstorm last night. In the morning, the driveway was filled with snow. I put on my coat and said, "I'm going to *shovel snow.*"

4. Tracking. The story from Session Seven is tracked again. This time, a second paragraph is added to the story. A copy of the story is not given to

the client. The client is asked to track the story, first V-only, then A-only, and finally AV.

Last spring, a pedestrian bridge was built in our town. It was built across the river. The river runs through the town. I enjoy walking across the bridge. Canada geese nest on the shores of the river. You can see lots of geese when you walk over the bridge.

The bridge was built by volunteers. The volunteers came from all over North America. The bridge is built of wood and is held together with pegs. Not one nail was put into the bridge. The bridge is an attractive addition to the landscape of our town.

SESSION NINE

1. The client is presented with a sentence AV. One word in the sentence is V-only. The client is asked to fill in this word using the context of the sentence.

    a. How was _____?
    b. May I borrow your _____?
    c. The _____ won't work.
    d. Did you hear about the _____?
    e. What is a _____?
    f. We saw a _____?
    g. Didn't you know about _____?
    h. He doesn't like to _____?
    i. We couldn't find the _____?
    j. Around the corner is a _____?

2. A story is presented. The first sentence is presented, and the sentences that follow are added one at a time until all of the sentences are presented in succession. The client is asked to repeat the sentences as presented by the practitioner. The sentences are first presented V-only, then A-only, and finally AV.

    Yesterday I went to the store.
    I had to buy groceries.
    When I arrived at the store, I couldn't find a grocery cart.
    I had to carry all my groceries in my arms.
    Soon, my arms were getting sore.
    A young man approached me.
    He had an empty grocery cart.
    He had found the cart outside.
    He gave me the empty cart.
    I was pleased to have the cart.
    I thanked the young man.

3. AV short story. The last sentence of the story is presented in print to the client. Some of the words of the last sentence are left out. The practitioner presents the last sentence V-only, and the client is asked to fill in the missing words. If the words cannot be filled in, the sentence is presented A-only and then AV.

    a. My mother and I were downtown shopping. It was Saturday morning and the streets were filled with cars. We were waiting to cross the street. I commented, "The *street* is filled with *cars.*"
    b. I like to read the newspaper while I eat breakfast. The other morning, my husband was trying to tell me something while I was reading. After I didn't respond, he said, "Will you please *Put down* that *paper!*"
    c. The other day, I decided to hang a mirror in the hallway. The mirror was heavy and slipped out of my hands. The mirror fell to the floor and broke. I said, "That's *seven years* of *bad luck* for me!"
    d. Yesterday, I went to a baseball game. In the third inning, there were three players on base. The player at bat hit the ball. I said, "I *hope* it's a *home run!*"
    e. He likes sugar in his coffee. In fact he likes three lumps of sugar in each cup. One day, our coffee cups were switched. I took one sip and said, "This *isn't* my *coffee!*"
    f. We went out to a restaurant for dinner last night. I ordered a baked potato with my meal. The waiter asked me, "Would you like *butter* and *sour cream?*"
    g. Fall is my favorite season. I love to see the leaves change color. It is sad when the leaves fall off the trees. After a wind storm, I know I'll be saying, "I'd better *rake* the *leaves.*"
    h. Sometimes I eat lunch on the run. My favorite fast lunch is a hot dog. I go to the stand and order the hot dog. The vendor asks me, "Would you like *mustard* and *relish?*"
    i. We decided to paint our living room. While painting the ceiling, some paint started to drip on me. I was told, "You have *paint* in your *hair.*"
    j. I was sitting and watching television. I thought I heard a knocking sound. I said, "I think *someone* is *at* the *door.*"

SESSION TEN

1. Story activity. The first sentence is presented and then the sentences that follow are added one at a time until all of the sentences are presented in succession. The client is asked to repeat the sentences as presented by the practitioner. The sentences are first presented V-only, then A-only, and finally AV.

Bill Jones loves to cross-country ski.
For Christmas, he bought cross-country skis for himself and his wife.
There was no snow until Christmas day.
On Christmas morning, the Joneses woke up to a blizzard.
It snowed enough that they were able to ski on Boxing Day.
The cross-country skis turned out to be the perfect Christmas present.

2. Story tracking. First, key words are presented V-only, A-only, and then AV. The client is asked to identify each key word. Second, sentences that contain the key words are presented to the client. The sentences are presented V-only, A-only, and then AV. The client is asked to repeat each sentence verbatim. Finally, a story is presented to the client. The client is asked to track the story, V-only, A-only, and then AV.

plant	vegetable	garden
eaten	dessert	grow
squash	butternut	Hubbard
course	turban	spaghetti
zucchini	summer	baked
stored	cool	cooked
frozen	custard	use

a. I like to grow squash.
b. I have a vegetable garden.
c. There are many varieties of squash.
d. Squash can be stored easily.
e. You can eat squash as a main course or a dessert.

Every year we plant a large vegetable garden in the backyard. We grow many kinds of vegetables.

I think that squash are easy to grow. I have grown butternut, Hubbard, turban, spaghetti, zucchini, and summer squash.

Squash can be stored in a cool area for long periods of time. Squash can also be cooked and frozen for later use. Squash can be eaten as part of a main course or baked in a custard or pie for dessert. Squash is a versatile vegetable.

3. Story tracking. The procedures from the previous tracking story are followed.

birdfeeder	backyard	attracts
types	birdseed	blue jays
cardinals	chickadees	finches
doves	squirrels	clothesline
suspended	discourage	climb
difficulty	feet	down

a. The birdfeeder attracts many birds.
b. The birdfeeder also attracts squirrels.
c. Our birdfeeder is suspended from our clothesline.
d. The birdfeeder is filled with birdseed.
e. The squirrels eat the birdseed quickly.

We have a birdfeeder in our backyard. It attracts many different types of birds.

Once the feeder is filled with birdseed, the birds soon arrive. I have seen blue jays, cardinals, chickadees, finches, and doves at the feeder.

The birdfeeder also attracts squirrels. We suspended the feeder from the clothesline about six feet from our house to discourage the squirrels. The squirrels climb along the clothesline and suspend themselves down to the feeder with very little difficulty.

The birdseed disappears quickly once the squirrels arrive.

SESSION ELEVEN

1. A sentence is presented AV with one word missing. The client is asked to fill in the missing word using the sentence context.

a. _____ will not _____.
b. I _____ the _____.
c. Any _____ will _____.
d. Do not _____ _____.
e. The _____ is _____.
f. There isn't _____ _____.
g. Do you _____ _____?
h. They will _____ _____.
i. _____ didn't want _____.
j. Put the _____ _____.

2. Story activity. The first sentence is presented, and the sentences that follow are added one at a time until all the sentences are presented in succession. The client is asked to repeat the sentences as presented by the practitioner. The sentences are first presented V-only, then A-only, and finally AV.

John received a pair of hockey skates for his birthday.
This was the first pair of skates he has ever had.
John's parents took him to the rink.
They intended to teach him how to skate.
Once John put the skates on he ventured out onto the rink.
He spent most of the time falling down and getting back up.
At the end of his first lesson, John was able to stand on his own.
By the end of the third lesson, he was able to skate on his own.

3. Story tracking

lemon balm	bushy	plant
green	pot	relaxing
backyard	scent	mint
attract	water	honey
bees	soups	sauces
salads	steep	fish
tea handful	rinse	
soothing		

   a. Lemon balm grows in my backyard.
   b. Lemon balm has light green leaves.
   c. Lemon balm can be used to flavor foods.
   d. You can make tea with lemon balm leaves.
   e. Lemon balm attracts bees.

Lemon balm is a bushy plant with light green leaves. I have a lemon balm plant in my backyard. The leaves have a lemon scent and lemon-mint flavored leaves that attract bees. I use lemon balm leaves in soups, sauces, and salads and with fish. My favorite use of lemon balm is in tea. I pick a handful of leaves, rinse them, and put them in a pot. I pour boiling water over the leaves and let the tea steep for ten minutes. The tea has a lemony taste and is very soothing and relaxing. It is very tasty with a teaspoon of honey.

SESSION TWELVE

1. A sentence is presented AV with one word missing. The client is asked to fill in the missing word, using context sentences.

   a. If you _____ I'll _____.
   b. You can often _____ _____.
   c. All _____ _____ must _____.
   d. What _____ you _____ _____?
   e. _____ _____ about your _____?
   f. _____ to the _____ _____.
   g. Many _____ like to _____.
   h. Did you _____ to _____?
   i. Try to _____ at _____.
   j. _____ and the _____ _____.

2. Story tracking

driving	work	windshield
cracked	a.m.	highway
trucks	gravel	flew
hit	damage	done
license	noticed	round

spot	side	drop
water	chipped	cold
heater	yesterday	replaced
bill	taken	

a. I leave for work at 7:30 a.m.
b. I drive to work every morning.
c. There are many large trucks on the highway.
d. Gravel flew up and hit my windshield.
e. The crack in the windshield spread.
f. I had the windshield replaced.

Last week, when I was driving to work, my windshield was cracked. I left for work at 7:30 a.m. and was driving along the highway. There are always a lot of large trucks on the highway. One truck was coming toward me, and gravel flew up and hit my windshield. At the time, it didn't look as if any damage had been done. When I arrived at work, I noticed a small, round spot on the driver's side of the windshield. It almost looked like a drop of water. The windshield had been chipped.

With all the cold weather over the week, I had to use the heater in the car. A crack appeared out of the chip in the windshield. Soon the crack worked its way farther up and down the windshield.

Yesterday, I took the car in to have the windshield replaced. When I saw the bill, I wished I had taken down the license number of the truck!

3. Scripted conversation. The client is given only the script for his or her part in the conversation. The client is instructed to read his or her part aloud, one line at a time. The practitioner presents a response, V-only, and the client is asked to repeat the response. If the response cannot be repeated, it is presented A-only and finally AV.

Client
1. No one writes letters anymore!
2. Don't you think that people lose touch with each other when they don't write?
3. I can't afford to be calling all my friends.
4. Yes, I do, and I quite enjoy writing letters.

Practitioner
1. Well, it doesn't bother me because I don't like writing letters.
2. Not really. I call my friends regularly on the phone.
3. Do you still write letters?
4. Well, I'm glad you enjoy it!

SESSION THIRTEEN

1. The client is presented with a sentence AV with one word missing. The client is asked to fill in the missing word by using the context of the sentence.

    a. I'm so _____ I could _____.
    b. Didn't you _____ I _____ _____?
    c. Most _____ will _____ to _____.
    d. I tried to _____ _____ _____.
    e. My _____ was _____ _____ _____.
    f. Do you _____ a _____ _____?
    g. What _____ is your _____ _____?
    h. I _____ to _____ my _____.
    i. She _____ her _____ every _____.
    j. The _____ _____ was not _____.

2. Story tracking

moved	home	ago
boxes	garage	storage
belongings	still	weekend
root	junk	accumulate
wood	doors	light
fixtures	bricks	find
Christmas	decorations	unpacking
sale		

    a. We moved to a new home six months ago.
    b. We stored a lot of our boxes in the garage.
    c. We have collected a lot of junk.
    d. We can't find any of the things we need.
    e. We couldn't find our Christmas decorations.
    f. We should have a garage sale.

    When we moved to our new home six months ago, a lot of our boxes were put into the garage for storage. We had to plan where we wanted our belongings to go. Unfortunately, a lot of the boxes are still in the garage.

    Every weekend we go out to the garage and root through the boxes. It is unbelievable how much junk you can accumulate. We have pieces of wood, old doors, old light fixtures, bricks—you name it and it's probably stored in our garage!

    The problem is that there are things that we need stored in the garage, but we can't find them! At Christmas we couldn't find any of our decorations, but we know they are somewhere in the garage!

    Once we finish unpacking the boxes, we may have to have a garage sale!

3. Scripted conversation

Client	Practitioner
1. Hello, Bob. Imagine meeting you in the grocery store.	1. Hello, Frank.
2. I'm looking for some nice ripe tomatoes. Have you seen any?	2. I think I saw some over there. What do you think of these prices?
3. It's ridiculous how much things cost these days!	3. I couldn't agree with you more. I'm lucky I don't have a family to feed!
4. Have all your children left home?	4. Yes, the last of them moved out about a year ago. What about you?
5. I still have one at home and he eats like a horse!	5. You must really be affected when grocery prices keep rising.
6. I sure am!	

SESSION FOURTEEN

1. Story tracking

dinners	chance	together
tries	least	appetizers
year	country	catch
doing	generation	desserts
growing	rent	hall
time	group	compile
contribute	dish	feed
casseroles	salads	recipes
cookbook	passed	future

  a. We have a family dinner at least once a year.
  b. People come from all over the country for our family dinners.
  c. People get to know the new generation of the family.
  d. Our family keeps growing.
  e. You need a lot of food to feed our family.
  f. We could write a family cookbook.

Family dinners give you a good chance to get the whole family together. Our family tries to get together at least once a year. People come from all over the country to get together.

A family dinner gives you the chance to catch up on what people have been doing. It gives everyone the chance to see and get to know the new generation of the family.

Sometimes we have as many as thirty people at dinner. If the family keeps growing, we may have to rent a hall!

It takes a long time to prepare food for a large group. Lately, we have asked everyone to contribute one dish per family. Each dish should feed about four people. People bring casseroles, salads, appetizers, and desserts.

One of these days, we should compile our recipes into a family cookbook that could be passed to future generations.

2.   Scripted conversation

Client	**Practitioner**
1. Hi, Bill.	1. Hi, George.
2. How are you?	2. I'm fine. How are you?
3. Pretty good. How are the grandchildren?	3. They're growing like weeds!
4. I love it when my grandchildren come to visit.	4. So do I, but I also like it when they go home!
5. How many grandchildren do you have?	5. An even dozen. How about you?
6. I have two.	6. It'd be quieter at your house than at mine!

SESSION FIFTEEN

1.   Story tracking

newspaper	route	son
started	job	weeks
a.m.	p.m.	delivered
door	day	flyers
takes	minutes	load
bags	houses	carries
returns	empty	bad
longer	chased	dog
play		

a.   My son started delivering papers two weeks ago.
b.   The papers arrive at our house at 9:30 a.m.
c.   The papers must be delivered before 5:00 p.m.
d.   It takes about thirty minutes to put the flyers in the papers.
e.   There are 150 houses on the route.
f.   The route takes about three hours.
g.   Sometimes dogs chase my son.

My son has a paper route. He just started the job two weeks ago. At about 9:30 a.m. the papers are delivered to our front door. They must all be delivered before 5:00 p.m. the same day.

I help my son place the flyers in each newspaper. This takes us about thirty minutes. We then load the papers into bags.

My son has 150 houses on his route. He carries only one bag of papers with him at a time. He returns to pick up a new bag once the old bag is empty.

It takes my son about three hours to deliver all the papers. If the weather is bad, it takes him a bit longer.

One day when my son was delivering his papers, he was chased by a dog. Thank goodness the dog only wanted to play!

2. Scripted conversation

Client	**Practitioner**
1. Hi, Linda.	1. Hi, Pam.
2. Do you still drive your car?	2. No, I've stopped recently and am taking the bus.
3. Why did you decide to stop driving?	3. Because there are so many crazy drivers on the road.
4. I agree.	4. I can't stand it when they weave in and out of the lanes.
5. That bothers me too.	5. Those people are never involved in accidents; they just cause them.
6. Yes, I agree. Are you going to sell your car?	6. No, I'm keeping it for emergency purposes.
7. That sounds like a wise idea to me.	

SESSION SIXTEEN

1. Story tracking

dogs	breed	beagle
nose	walk	ground
hits	funny	snow
using	shovel	end
trailed	squirrel	minutes
keen	sense	smell
hunting	rabbits	hares
trained	detect	plants
airports	sniffing	banned

a. My favorite breed of dog is the beagle.
b. Beagles have an excellent sense of smell.
c. Beagles make good hunting dogs.
d. I have heard that beagles can be trained to detect plants.

e. Beagles can help sniff out plant materials that are banned from being imported into the country.

I am a dog lover. My favorite breed is the beagle. The only problem with a beagle is his nose!

As soon as you take a beagle outside for a walk, his nose hits the ground. It is funny to watch a beagle in the snow, because it looks like he is using his nose as a shovel!

If you let a beagle follow his nose, you could end up anywhere. Once we trailed after a squirrel for ten minutes. The beagle's keen sense of smell makes it a good hunting dog. It is good for trailing rabbits and hares.

I have heard that beagles can be trained to detect plants. Beagles can be helpful at the airports, sniffing out plant material that is banned from being imported into the country.

2. Scripted conversation

Client	Practitioner
1. Hello, Marge.	1. Oh, hello, Betty.
2. How are you?	2. I'm just fine. How are you?
3. I'm fine. I'd like to invite you to come to a New Year's party.	3. I'd love to!
4. Great! It wouldn't be a party without you!	4. Well thanks! Can I bring anything?
5. Sure, could you bring some snack food?	5. Yes. How about some potato chips and dip?
6. You always make such wonderful dip!	6. Thanks! I think I'll bring the dip that's loaded with garlic.
7. Great, that's my favorite.	7. What time should I be there?
8. Come around 7:30 and we can chat while I get things organized.	8. I always like to be the first to arrive!
9. I'll see you around 7:30.	9. Yes. Bye for now.
10. Bye.	

SESSION SEVENTEEN

1. Story tracking

year	concern	raised
harmful	ultraviolet	sun
rays	exposed	thinning
ozone	daily	unprotected

skin	damage	done
screen	best	covered
outside	wear	shirts
pants	hats	

a. People are being exposed to harmful ultraviolet sun rays.
b. Higher levels of harmful sun rays are penetrating the ozone layer.
c. There are daily reports on the levels of harmful sun rays.
d. Sunscreen can help protect you from harmful sun rays.
e. Keeping your skin covered while in the sun is a good idea.

Over the past year, concern has been raised over the amount of harmful ultraviolet sun rays that people are being exposed to. With the thinning of the ozone layer, people are being exposed to higher levels of harmful sun rays. Daily reports are now made on the levels of ultraviolet rays. These reports tell you how long unprotected skin can be exposed before damage is done. One way to protect ourselves from these harmful rays is to use sunscreen. The best way to protect yourself is to keep your skin covered. Some people who work outside every day wear long-sleeved shirts, pants, and hats.

2. Conversation practice. A topic is introduced by the practitioner. The practitioner encourages the client to express his or her views and makes comments during the conversation. The conversation is carried out AV. Background noise can be introduced during the conversation to add difficulty. The practitioner encourages the client to use the following strategies during the conversation when information is missed. First, the client asks the speaker to repeat the segment that was missed. Second, the client asks the speaker to rephrase the segment that was missed. Third, the client asks a question that might help fill in the missing information. Finally, the client asks for the topic or key word. If the client is unaware that some of the information has been misinterpreted or missed, the speaker repeats the missed information.

Topic: Television

Practitioner's Opening Statement   I used to enjoy watching television, but I don't seem to watch it very much lately.

Comments for the Practitioner to Use to Help Keep the Conversation Going
a. My favorite programs are comedies. I especially enjoy Topo Gigio.
b. There is too much violence on television these days.
c. I read somewhere that people don't read as much these days, so television is important for relaying information.
d. There are special assistive listening devices that you can use with the television, such as FM systems and infrared systems.

e. Closed captioning is important for people who can't hear the television.
f. I often watch a channel dedicated to the weather so I know what the weather is like.
g. My family loves sports and likes to watch the channel dedicated to sports.

SESSION EIGHTEEN

1. Story tracking

beekeeping	apiculture	profitable
hobby	combs	spring
buy	supplier	queen
wood	starve	casing
workers	drones	dot
back	hive	sugar
solution	forage	nectar
pollen	collected	escape
board	upper	layers

a. The proper term for beekeeping is apiculture.
b. The queen bee has a dot on her back.
c. You begin working with bees in the spring.
d. Bees should be supplied with a sugar and water solution.
e. Bees must be moved out of the hive before you collect the honey.
f. A bee-escape board can be used to move the bees.

The proper term for beekeeping is apiculture. Apiculture can be an interesting and profitable hobby.

If you are new to apiculture, you begin your work in the spring. You should buy your bees from a reputable supplier. The bees will be in a box. The queen is kept in a wood casing and is separated from the workers and drones. The queen has a dot on her back so that she can be easily identified.

Once you get the bees, they must be put into a hive. They should be supplied with a sugar and water solution until they are able to forage for nectar and pollen from the spring flowers.

The bees should be checked once a week until the honey is ready to be collected. Bees must be moved out of the hive before you can collect the honey. A bee-escape board can be used to move the bees to the lower levels of the hive, so that the upper layers can be removed. Once this is done, the honey can be collected. Some full combs of honey should be left in the hive so that the bees do not starve over the winter.

2.   Conversation practice

Topic: Snow Storms

Practitioner's Opening Statement   This year has been a record year for the number of snow storms.

Comments for the Practitioner to Use to Help Keep the Conversation Going
a.   Some days, none of the school buses were running.
b.   There have been many bad accidents on the roads.
c.   The trains always seem to make it through the storms.
d.   Just as you finish shoveling, the plow comes along and blocks the driveway.
e.   I remember when I was young and I listened to the radio, hoping to hear that school was canceled.

SESSION NINETEEN

1.   Story tracking

cat	fact	content
living	indoors	adapt
city	country	interesting
breeds	Burmese	Rex
Himalayan	Persian	Siamese
companions	therapy	nursing
pets	residents	Humane societies
body	language	tails
ears	feelings	

a.   Cats are a popular pet.
b.   Cats can live indoors or outdoors.
c.   Some interesting breeds of cat include Burmese, Rex, Himalayan, Persian, and Siamese.
d.   Sometimes cats are brought to nursing homes to visit the residents.
e.   Cats use body language to communicate their feelings.

A lot of people are cat lovers. In fact, cats are a very popular pet.
Cats are often content living indoors. Cats adapt well to life in the city or in the country.
There are many interesting breeds of cat, including Burmese, Rex, Himalayan, Persian, and Siamese.
Cats make good companions, and many people believe that it can be good therapy to live with a cat.
Some nursing homes keep cats as pets for residents. They also have humane societies come in with cats and other animals for visits.
Cats have their own body language. They use their tails, ears, and voice to communicate their feelings.

2.   Conversation practice

Topic: Computers

Practitioner's Opening Statement   Everyone seems to rely on computers these days.

Comments for the Practitioner to Use to Help Keep the Conversation Going
a.   I was at the bank the other day and the computers were down, so they couldn't update my passbook.
b.   A friend of mine did a whole day's work on her computer and then lost all her work because she forgot to tell the computer to save it.
c.   I never thought I would use a computer, but now that I'm used to it I find it invaluable.
d.   I can type faster on the computer keyboard than on a typewriter.
e.   It is easier to correct mistakes and edit your work on a computer.

SESSION TWENTY

1.   Story tracking

watch	movies	actresses
Gloria Swanson	Greta Garbo	Bette Davis
role	aging	*Sunset Boulevard*
star	*Ninotchka*	amusing
gentleman	Eiffel Tower	trade
envoys	portrayal	*All About Eve*
height	career	

a.   My favorite movie actresses are Gloria Swanson, Greta Garbo, and Bette Davis.
b.   I have seen the movie *Sunset Boulevard* many times.
c.   My favorite movie with Greta Garbo is *Ninotchka.*
d.   Greta Garbo meets a gentleman at the Eiffel Tower.
e.   Bette Davis gives a wonderful performance in *All About Eve.*

I love to watch movies. My favorite movie actresses are Gloria Swanson, Greta Garbo, and Bette Davis.

I have seen the movie *Sunset Boulevard* many times. Gloria Swanson is wonderful in her role as an aging movie star.

My favorite movie with Greta Garbo is *Ninotchka.* This movie from the 1930s is very amusing. My favorite scene is when Garbo meets the gentleman at the Eiffel Tower. The three trade envoys she is sent to check up on are also very amusing.

Bette Davis has many great performances, but my favorite is her performance in *All About Eve.* She is wonderful in her portrayal of a woman at the height of her career.

2. Conversation practice

Topic: Vacations

Practitioner's Opening Statement I haven't been on a vacation in years.

Comments for the Practitioner to Use to Help Keep the Conversation Going
a. A lot of people go to Florida every winter.
b. Vacations can be expensive.
c. I would love to go to Europe. Have you ever been there?
d. I always pack too many clothes when I go away.
e. I don't like waiting around in airports.

SESSION TWENTY-ONE

1. Story tracking

dinner	try	limit
eating	Indian	lentils
aromatic	restaurants	expensive
different	types	food
cuisine	fruits	stomach
Chinese	spring rolls	vermicelli
mixed	corner	tandoori
nuts	oyster	Greek
moussaka	souvlaki	excellent
basmati	delicate	yogurt

a. I go out to dinner once a week.
b. Eating at restaurants can be expensive.
c. I enjoy eating Chinese food.
d. There is an excellent Greek restaurant in my neighborhood.
e. Indian food is my favorite cuisine.
f. Talking about food makes my stomach rumble.

   I like to go out to dinner. I try to limit myself to going out once a week because eating out at restaurants can be expensive.
   I like to try different types of food. Chinese food is one of my favorites. I love spring rolls, vermicelli noodles with ginger, lemon chicken, and mixed vegetables in oyster sauce.
   I also enjoy Greek food. The thought of moussaka, lamb souvlaki, and salad makes my mouth water. There is an excellent Greek restaurant just around the corner from where I live.
   By far my favorite is Indian cuisine. I love tandoori chicken, basmati rice, and the delicate mixtures of vegetables, lentils, fruits, and nuts in yogurt with aromatic spices.
   Talking about all this lovely food is making my stomach rumble!

2. Conversation practice

Topic: Weddings

Practitioner's Opening Statement   Weddings cost a lot of money. I guess that is why a lot of people are having small weddings these days.

Comments for the Practitioner to Use to Help Keep the Conversation Going
a.   You usually see people you haven't seen for years at weddings.
b.   I usually eat too much at weddings.
c.   Have you ever watched any royal weddings on television?
d.   It seems like cameras are always snapping at weddings.
e.   These days, people often videotape their weddings.

SESSION TWENTY-TWO

1. Story tracking

Italy	interesting	Vatican City
country	Sorrento	Capri
Rome	Colosseum	center
city	A.D.	entertained
gladiators	fought	beasts
Forum	commercial	political
several	contains	historic
tombs	temples	Pantheon
monument	gods	complete
building		

a.   Rome, Sorrento, and Capri are all places in Italy.
b.   Vatican City is a country within Italy.
c.   The Colosseum is in Rome.
d.   There are many things to see in the Roman Forum.
e.   The Pantheon is a monument dedicated to the Roman Gods.

Italy is an interesting country to visit. I have been to Italy and visited Sorrento, Capri, and Rome. I have also visited Vatican City.

If you stay in Rome, there are many things to see. The Colosseum is near the center of the city. It was completed in 80 A.D. and could accommodate 50,000 people. In the Colosseum, people were entertained by gladiators who fought each other and fought wild beasts.

The Roman Forum was a center of commercial, religious, and political life. The Roman Forum is the oldest of several forums and contains many historic tombs and temples.

Another important place to visit is the Pantheon. It is a monument dedicated to all the Roman gods. It is the most complete building remaining from the time period in which it was built.

2.   Conversation practice

Topic: Birthdays

Practitioner's Opening Statement   Some people don't like you to remember their birthdays.

Comments for the Practitioner to Use to Help Keep the Conversation Going
a.   When I was growing up I used to have big birthday parties.
b.   My favorite birthday cake is a chocolate cake.
c.   It's embarrassing when they put a sparkler on the top of a cake when you go out to a restaurant to celebrate.
d.   We used to wear party hats at birthday parties.
e.   I usually take my friends out for dinner for their birthdays.

SESSION TWENTY-THREE

1.   Story tracking

island	Toronto	Canada
ferry	city	Algonquin
Centre	Forestry	Mugg's
Olympic	Snake	South
Wards	years	close-knit
parkland	metro	residents
fought	won	right
mainland	groceries	supplies
summer	days	picnics
lying	beaches	Hanlan's Point
amusement	boasts	kilometer
boardwalk		

a.   Toronto Island is in Lake Ontario.
b.   The island is a short ferry ride from the city of Toronto, Ontario, Canada.
c.   There are eight islands that make up Toronto Island.
d.   People live on Toronto Island and people like to visit the island in the summer.
e.   People have picnics, lie on the beach, and visit the amusement park.

Just a short ferry ride across Lake Ontario from the city of Toronto, Ontario, Canada, lies Toronto Island.
Eight islands make up Toronto Island. These include Algonquin Island, Centre Island, Forestry Island, Mugg's Island, Olympic Island, Snake Island, South Island, and Wards Island.

People have lived on the island for many years, and it is a close-knit community. Metro Toronto had wanted to remove all homes from the island and turn it into parkland. The residents have fought to keep their homes and have recently won that right.

People who live on the island must go to the mainland for groceries and other supplies.

People from the mainland enjoy spending summer days on the island having picnics, lying on the beaches at Hanlan's Point, or visiting the Centre Island Amusement Park. The island also boasts a two-kilometer-long board-walk.

2. Conversation practice

Topic: Baking

Practitioner's Opening Statement   For as long as I can remember, I have enjoyed baking.

Comments for the Practitioner to Use to Help Keep the Conversation Going
a. My mother and grandmother were excellent bakers.
b. I am nervous about working with yeast. Have you ever baked using yeast?
c. It is a lot easier to buy baked goods from a store.
d. We have an excellent bakery in our town.
e. I love homemade bread, fresh out of the oven.

SESSION TWENTY-FOUR

1. Story tracking

Pompeii	town	Italy
destroyed	volcano	semicircles
skyline	Mount Vesuvius	erupted
excavated	streets	shops
bustling	sitting	paintings
mosaics	villa	theater
terraced	concentric	dominates

a. Pompeii is a town in Italy.
b. Pompeii was destroyed when a volcano erupted.
c. The town has been excavated.
d. There are paintings and mosaics in the houses.
e. The large theater has terraced seating.
f. You can see Mount Vesuvius from Pompeii.

Have you ever visited Pompeii? It is a very interesting place to visit.

Pompeii is a town in Italy that was destroyed when a volcano, Mount Vesuvius, erupted.

The town has been excavated, and there are many things to see. You can walk down the streets and see the shops that were bustling with people long ago.

Many paintings and mosaics can be viewed on the walls of villas.

The large theater is very impressive. The seating is terraced and is formed into concentric semicircles. One can only imagine sitting and watching the entertainment that was available long ago.

The once-destructive Mount Vesuvius dominates the skyline of the town of Pompeii.

2. Conversation practice

Topic: Stamps

Practitioner's Opening Statement   A lot of people like to collect stamps.

Comments for the Practitioner to Use to Help Keep the Conversation Going
a. People who study and collect stamps are called philatelists.
b. Many famous people have had their pictures on stamps.
c. I saw a stamp from the United States with a picture of Elvis Presley on it.
d. In Canada, a lot of stamps have a picture of Queen Elizabeth II on them.
e. Sometimes stamps go through the mail and are not postmarked.

SUGGESTED ACTIVITIES FOR CARRYOVER

Having a client and his or her significant others work together at home helps them to communicate more effectively. Suggested activities for home study can include the following materials used in the V-only, A-only, and AV conditions: newspaper articles, magazine articles, comic strips, recipes, crossword puzzles, short stories, poems, and books.

REFERENCES

De Filippo, C.L. (1988). Tracking for speechreading training. *Volta Review, 90,* 215–239.

Erber, N.P. (1988). *Communication therapy for hearing-impaired adults.* Abbotsford: Clavis.

Haug, O., & Haug. S. (1977). *Help for the hard-of-hearing: A speech reading and auditory training manual for home and professionally guided training.* Springfield: Thomas.

Jeffers, J., & Barley, M. (1979). *Look, now hear this: Combined auditory training and speechreading instruction.* Springfield: Thomas.

Jennings, M.B., Sheppard, A., & Sutherland, G. (1991). *Aural rehabilitation curriculum series: Hearing help class one—Help for hearing aid users.* Toronto: Canadian Hearing Society.

Mecklenburg, D.J., Dowell, R.C., & Jenison, V.W. (1987). *Mini-system 22: Cochlear implant rehabilitation manual.* Englewood: Cochlear Corporation.

Pichora-Fuller, M.K., & Robertson, L.F. (1993). Evaluation of a hearing rehabilitation program in a home for the aged. Presented at the Academy of Rehabilitative Audiology Summer Institute, June 10-13, 1993, Howey-in-the-Hills, Florida.

Walther, E.F. (1982). *Lipreading.* Chicago: Nelson-Hall.

Windle, J., & Stout, G. (1992). *Developmental approach to successful listening: DASL II.* Englewood: Resource Point.

Author Index

Subject Index